The Epidemic of Coronary Heart Disease in South Asian Populations: Causes and Consequences

First Edition

Edited by

Kiran C R Patel

Chairman of Trustees, South Asian Health Foundation, UK

and University Dept of Cardiology, Birmingham

Raj S Bhopal CBE

Bruce and John Usher Chair of Public Health, University of Edinburgh, UK

Patron, South Asian Health Foundation, UK

Distributed by :

South Asian Health Foundation

26 Lightwoods Hill

Bearwood

Birmingham B67 5EA

British Library Cataloguing in Publication Data:

Available on request

ISBN   0-9546712-0-1

Publisher: South Asian Health Foundation

Project manager: Rumeena Gujral

Design of cover: Shahid Zaman

Contents

List of Contributors

C Agyemang, Erasmus Medical Centre, Department of Health Policy and Management, Erasmus University of Rotterdam, Rotterdam, The Netherlands

M Banerjee, Clinical Epidemiology Group, Unit of Chronic Disease Epidemiology, University of Manchester Medical School, Manchester

R S Bhopal, Community Health Sciences, College of Medicine and Veterinary Medicine, University of Edinburgh, Edinburgh, and Patron, South Asian Health Foundation

J C Chambers, National Heart and Lung Institute, Imperial College School of Medicine, Hammersmith Hospital, London

J Kennedy Cruickshank, Clinical Epidemiology Group, Unit of Chronic Disease Epidemiology, University of Manchester Medical School, and Consultant Physician Diabetes and Hypertension, Manchester Royal Infirmary, Manchester

C Fall, Medical Research Council Environmental Epidemiology Unit, University of Southampton, Southampton

S Gupta, Department of Cardiology, Whipps Cross and St Bartholomew's Hospitals, Leytonstone, London

S Harding, Medical Research Council Social and Public Health Sciences Unit, University of Glasgow, Glasgow

M T Kearney, Department of Cardiology, Guy's, King's and St. Thomas' School of Medicine, King's College London, London

J Kooner, National Heart and Lung Institute, Imperial College School of Medicine, Hammersmith Hospital, London

M Marmot, International Centre for Health and Society, Department of Epidemiology and Public Health, University College London, London

J C Oldroyd, Clinical Epidemiology Group, Unit of Chronic Disease Epidemiology, University of Manchester Medical School, Manchester

N J Samani, Department of Cardiovascular Sciences, University of Leicester, Leicester

T A B Sanders, Nutrition Food and Health Research Centre, Franklin-Wilkins Building, King's College London, London

A M Shah, Department of Cardiology, Guy's, King's and St. Thomas' School of Medicine, King's College London, London, and Patron, South Asian Health Foundation

P Sharma, Clinical Pharmacology Unit, University of Cambridge, and Trustee, South Asian Health Foundation

A Vyas, Clinical Epidemiology Group, Unit of Chronic Disease Epidemiology, University of Manchester Medical School, Manchester

M White, School of Health Sciences, University of Newcastle Medical School, Newcastle upon Tyne

R Williams, Medical Research Council Social and Public Health Sciences Unit, University of Glasgow, Glasgow

Q Zaidi, British Heart Foundation, London

Foreword

The study of the health and disease of populations after migration has a long tradition in epidemiology. The communities with birth or ancestral origins in the Indian subcontinent - now called South Asian - are a vital part of the social and economic fabric of modern, multicultural Britain. It is no surprise that, when exposed to a new environment and way of life, the health experience of South Asians, is different from that in their countries of origin. Their greater susceptibility to coronary heart disease is an important example, and was the subject of this ground-breaking symposium.

Coronary heart disease remains one of the leading killers in our country. Exploring the reasons for its even greater impact in South Asian communities living in Britain is an important area for research. Assessing the evidence to enable an effective public health response is a major challenge.

The symposium brought together leading researchers and thinkers in this field. They are to be congratulated for the quality of their contributions and, more than this, for their commitment to finding solutions to the problem of coronary heart disease in the South Asian communities living in Britain.

The publication will bring this important issue to a much wider audience and we believe enable many others to come forward to help advance understanding of the problem and action to combat it.

Professor Sir Liam Donaldson, Chief Medical Officer, on behalf of the Dept of Health
Professor Sir Charles George, on behalf of the British Heart Foundation
Lord Naren Patel, Patron, The South Asian Health Foundation

Preface

Coronary heart disease (CHD) poses a massive challenge globally. Over the last 50 years there has been an explosion of research from bench to bedside to population, to explore the multifactorial aetiology of CHD. One important discovery is that the UK population of South Asian origin is at significantly greater mortality risk from CHD than the population as a whole. Despite significant research the exact explanation(s) for the increased risk of South Asians is undetermined. In December 2001, The South Asian Health Foundation, with the support of the British Heart Foundation and the Department of Health hosted its first UK symposium on 'The epidemic of coronary heart disease in South Asian populations: causes and consequences.' Leading researchers in the field of ethnicity and coronary disease were invited to present their research and share knowledge to help in the management of this epidemic. This short monograph summarises and updates the work from the symposium, with an aim to disseminate this vital information. We are aware that this field is advancing rapidly but we hope, on behalf of The South Asian Health Foundation, that this monograph will highlight important and relevant issues to all involved in the management of South Asian patients with CHD. We would like to thank all of our contributors, the British Heart Foundation and Department of Health for their support in publication of this monograph and last but not least, the other Patrons and Trustees of the South Asian Health Foundation without whom the initial symposium and ensuing publication would not have been possible.

Kiran C R Patel

Raj S Bhopal

Acknowledgements

We would like to thank the authors who have provided exceptional contributions to this monograph and indeed, to the field of ethnicity and cardiovascular disease. Without their effort, progress in this field would be severely compromised. We also wish to thank the many individuals and bodies who have made this publication possible and the efforts of the SAHF Patrons and trustees. The BHF and Department of Health have provided funding towards this publication, which enables us to distribute to such a wide network. We also wish to thank Bristol Myers Squibb for sponsoring delegates to the original symposium in 2001.

The South Asian Health Foundation (UK)

The South Asian Health Foundation (registered. charity 1073178) was founded in 1999. It seeks to promote improvements in the quality of, and access to, health care and health promotion in South Asians; and to promote scholarship and research that leads to those objectives. Our work at a grass roots level includes community based meetings delivered throughout the UK in town halls, religious establishments and community centres (often bilingually). We are developing a national infrastructure to enable all South Asian communities to benefit equally and effectively from health promotion and educational advice, thus building upon the good work which already goes on in several areas and ensure that all South Asian communities benefit from these efforts. In 2001, we hosted the first UK symposium on ethnicity and CHD: "The epidemic of coronary heart disease in the South Asian populations: causes and consequences". The symposium brought together experts and researchers in the field of CHD in South Asians, to highlight current issues and facilitate collaboration for future research. The symposium has resulted in this monograph. Already working closely with the Department of Health and BHF, we are delighted to have become a member organisation of the National Heart Forum too.

Patrons and Trustees in December 2003 were:

Delegates of the Conference on 'The epidemic of coronary heart disease in South Asian populations: causes and consequences' London, December 2001

Lord Naren Patel	Patron, SAHF
Prof. Sir Liam Donaldson	Chief Medical Officer
Prof Sir Charles George	British Heart Foundation
Prof Sir Michael Marmot	University College London
Prof Waqar Ahmad	University of Leeds
Prof Raman Bedi	National Centre for Transcultural Oral Health
Prof Raj Bhopal	Patron, SAHF and University of Edinburgh
Prof K K Cheng	University of Birmingham
Prof Peter Elliot	Imperial College, London
Prof Jaspal Kooner	Imperial College, London
Prof Peter Macfarlane	University of Glasgow
Prof A Macgregor	St Georges Hospital, London
Prof M McCarthy	Imperial College, London
Prof Nilesh Samani	University of Leicester
Prof Tom Sanders	Kings College London, London
Prof James Scott	Imperial College, London
Prof Ajay Shah	Patron, SAHF and Kings College London, London
Prof Andrew Steptoe	University College London
Prof John Vann Jones	University of Bristol
Prof Peter Whincup	St Georges Hospital, London
Dr Charles Agyemang	University of Edinburgh
Dr Tariq Ali	Imperial College, London

Glossary

Glossary of terms relating to ethnicity and race used in this monograph are:

African
A person with African ancestral origins who self-identifies as African, but excluding South Asians.

Afro-Caribbean:
A person of African ancestral origins whose family settled in the Caribbean before coming to Britain and who self-identifies as Afro-Caribbean. (See also Black.)

Bangladeshi:
A person whose ancestry lies in the Indian subcontinent who self-identifies as Bangladeshi. (See also South Asian.)

Chinese:
A person with ancestral origins in China, including Hong Kong who self-identifies as Chinese.

Ethnicity[1]:
The social group a person belongs to, and both identifies with and is identified with, as a result of a mix of cultural and other factors including language, diet, religion, ancestry, and race. *See also race.*

European
Effectively this is a synonym for White (see below).

Indian:
A person whose ancestry lies in the Indian sub-continent who identifies as Indian (see, South Asian). (Major changes to India's geographical boundaries took place in 1947).

Pakistani:
A person whose ancestry lies in the Indian subcontinent who identifies as Pakistani (see South Asian).

Race: The group a person belongs to as a result of a mix of physical features (e.g. skin colour, hair texture), ancestry and geographical origins, as identified by others or, increasingly, as self identified. The importance of social factors in the creation and perpetuation of racial categories has led to the concept broadening to include social and political heritage, making its usage similar to ethnicity. Race and ethnicity are increasingly used as synonyms. *See also ethnicity.*

South Asian: A person whose ancestry is in the countries of the Indian sub-continent, including India, Pakistan, Bangladesh and Sri Lanka. (See also, Indian, Pakistani, Bangladeshi).

White: The term usually used to describe people with European ancestral origins who identify as white (sometimes called European, Caucasian or Caucasoid). The word is capitalised to highlight its specific use.

[1]The concepts of race and ethnicity are so intertwined that consideration of one necessarily requires consideration of the other. In this proposal the term ethnicity is used except when there is clear distinction between this and race.

1

Coronary heart disease in South Asians: The scale of the problem and the challenge

R S Bhopal

Introduction

In the 1950's and early 1960's, there emerged a gradual awareness that people with ancestral origins in the Indian subcontinent (henceforth called South Asians) are highly susceptible to cardiovascular diseases after migration to urban environments. Adelstein reported that in South Africa mortality rates for cardiovascular disease in Asian (mainly Indian) men and women, were much higher than in white men and women, respectively[1]. Such findings have been confirmed in several countries. In Britain, analysis of mortality rates around the censuses of 1971 by Marmot et al[2], 1981 by Balarajan et al[3] and 1991 by Wild and McKeigue[4] have shown a 15% - 60% excess in Indian Subcontinent born populations in comparison to the whole population of England and Wales. The validity of such data will be considered below but these data have confirmed the view that the cardiovascular diseases are the foremost killer of South Asians in Britain.

Coronary artery disease (CHD) is associated with industrialisation and modernisation of society. CHD was uncommon in Britain in the 19th century and when it became a major problem, the wealthy were affected more. Now CHD is the commonest cause of death and affects poorer people more. This time-trend has not been explained satisfactorily. While trends in South Asian populations remain unclear, there is some evidence of a decline in the absolute rates but an increase in the level of disparity in comparison to the whole population[3,5]; a result of rapidly declining rates in the white, European origin populations. The association between low social class and higher cardiovascular mortality and risk factors has emerged in South Asians[6,7,8].

CHD is still uncommon in many countries, particularly developing countries. There is a paucity of information on the frequency of CHD in the Indian subcontinent and seemingly it is uncommon in rural areas, but is a growing problem in the cities[9]. The epidemic in South Asians abroad forewarns of what may happen on the Indian Subcontinent.

Most middle aged and elderly British South Asians migrated here as young adults. Many came from rural or semi-urban areas at a time when CHD was not a common problem in India. There are two key questions about the rise of CHD in South Asians, first, why is the disease so unexpectedly common and, second, what can South Asians do to protect themselves?

The cause of CHD, despite massive research, remains unclear. There is a general agreement that the factors in box 1.1 increase risk of CHD either directly or indirectly. However, CHD occurs even without these risk factors. The roles of stress, racism, inflammation, infection, specific dietary constituents such as the B vitamins and folic acid, and environmental pollution and many other risk factors as causes of CHD remain unclear.

Box 1.1: Some key risk factors for CHD

Ageing

Male sex

A family history of heart disease

Economic deprivation

Smoking

High blood pressure

High concentrations of low density lipoprotein cholesterol and low concentration of high density lipoprotein cholesterol

Diabetes

Failing to exercise

A diet which promotes atheroma

The term South Asian, usually used to Indians, Pakistanis, Bangladeshis and sometimes Sri Lankans, defines many ethnic groups, with distinctive regions of origin, languages, religions and customs [10-13]. Language impacts in obvious ways on clinical care and health promotion. Religion governs important health behaviours such as taboos on smoking (Sikhs in particular), alcohol (Muslims in particular) and dietary customs. Social customs include taboos on smoking and drinking in women and chewing of tobacco, which is particularly common in Bangladeshis. The prevalence of current smoking in South Asians in Newcastle was 33% overall, but 14% in Indians, and 57% in Bangladeshis; and the prevalence of weekly aerobic activity was 22% overall, but 33% in Indians, 19% in Pakistanis and 14% in Bangladeshis[12]. Such heterogeneity is clearly important in CHD[10-13].

Since smoking is a major risk factor for CHD we would expect South Asians, Sikhs and Hindus to have lower CHD rates than average. However, the rates seem to be higher. This observation of a high CHD rate in South Asians, in the face of apparently lower prevalence of smoking and other major risk factors, and in the light of the low rate in the Indian Subcontinent, is a public health problem, one which is exciting and important for researchers. If the paradox can be explained we might gain more insight into the cause of CHD and refine strategies to prevent and control this disease in all populations.

Mortality data

Most data on CHD in UK ethnic groups come from mortality statistics, which have problems in coding cause of death, and rely upon country of birth as a marker of ethnicity reported by the informant, i.e., the person reporting the death. This may differ from that at census where country of birth is reported by the person completing the form. Mortality data are, mostly, reported by combining countries of birth e.g. India, Pakistan and Bangladesh as South Asian born, and many countries as Afro-Caribbean born[2-6, 10, 11]. This step has been taken in the attempt to iron out underlying errors in the data, and to boost numbers. Conclusions on CHD in South Asians combined are being readjusted in important ways by demonstration of differences between Indians, Pakistanis and Bangladeshis in both disease frequency (modest but important)[5] and coronary risk factors (substantial)[12, 13]. Despite these problems with

3

data quality, ethnic variations in CHD mortality in the United Kingdom are clearly substantial. Mortality rates in England and Wales around the 1991 census were 40 to 50% above average for ischaemic heart disease in South Asians in comparison to the total population. A summary of published data is in reference 10.

Table 1.1 summarises a reanalysis of data for 5 years around the 1991 census. Similar data are in Gill *et al*'s health needs assessment, where data on all major causes of death are available, for the age group 20 – 74 years[11]. Circulatory diseases, and specifically ischaemic heart disease, were the dominant causes of death in men and women. These SMRs corroborate past analyses showing these diseases as 30-50% more common compared to the population as a whole. The rates/100,000 for the 4 year period show that Indian men (3206/100,000) have much more circulatory disease than women (1469/100,000), a point obscured in SMR analyses. In Pakistani men, and to a lesser extent in women, circulatory diseases dominate. In women, the SMR for ischaemic heart disease was only 11% higher than in the whole population.

The number of deaths in Bangladeshi women was small, but neoplasms and circulatory diseases were the commonest cause of death. In women, CHD rates were relatively low in comparison to the whole population. This however, fits with earlier work by McKeigue (SMR for Bangladeshi women 108; Punjabis 206)[14], and by Balarajan (age standardised rate for Bangladeshi women 49, for Indians 98)[5] which is summarised in reference 10.

One common practice is combining Indians, Pakistanis, Bangladeshis and sometimes Sri Lankans and East Africans too into one category, South Asians. As Table 1.1 shows there are similarities and dissimilarities in mortality. Gill *et al* examined the data for Indians, Pakistanis, Bangladeshis and Sri Lankans as a single group of South Asians together and East Africans separately. They concluded that study of such a South Asian group is reasonable for diabetes, but not for many other causes[11]. Overall, it is probably wise to recognise the substantial heterogeneity in these populations' health needs even though the study of the separate groups poses additional challenges of smaller population size, and fewer deaths.

Table 1.1A: Mortality rates (1989-1992) for men for ischaemic heart disease by country of birth and sex for ages 45-74 years (unpublished analysis Wild S and Bhopal R)

Region of Birth	Number of deaths	Rate* per 100,000/4-years	SMR ** (95% CI)
India	2561	3206	141 (136, 147)
Pakistan	842	3062	144 (134, 154)
Bangladesh	366	3276	153 (137, 169)
China	99	1077	45 (37, 55)
Caribbean	816	1419	62 (58, 67)
W & S Africa	83	1301	56 (44, 69)
England and Wales	151953	1971	98 (98, 99)

Table 1.1B: Mortality rates (1989-1992) for women for ischaemic heart disease by country of birth and sex for ages 45-74 years (unpublished analysis Wild S and Bhopal R)

Region of Birth	Number of Deaths	Rate* per 100,000/4-years	SMR** (95%CI)
India	1020	1469	158 (149,168)
Pakistan	143	867	110 (93,130)
Bangladesh	26	509	94 (62, 138)
China	36	447	45 (31,62)
Caribbean	318	742	86 (77,96)
W & S Africa	20	757	67 (41, 104)
England and Wales	68810	739	99 (98, 99)

*Directly standardised to the population structure of England and Wales in 10 year age bands.

**Standardised mortality rates, with the population as a whole as the standard (100).

Arguably, the most important message from Table 1.1 is that CHD is not simply an inevitable consequence of migration – witness the extremely low rates of CHD in the Chinese.

Mortality data by ethnic group, as opposed to country of birth, are sparse, but early findings from the longitudinal survey are confirmatory in demonstrating that CHD is the dominant, and probably comparatively common, cause of death in South Asians. Some data are in Table 20 in Gill *et al's* report[11].

Morbidity data

Incidence data of high quality are not available, but some work on hospital morbidity in 'Asians' in Leicester[15] supports the mortality data. Information on prevalence of cardiovascular diseases from many local studies[10], and most recently the Health Survey for England '99, confirm that CHD (angina and heart attack) and stroke are very common - and the prevalence is higher than, or on a par with, that in the reference white or general populations. Table 1.2 is an extract of data from the Health Survey for England '99, on IHD and stroke combined. The point is to show the vast scale of the problem. About one-fifth of South Asian men and about one tenth of women report these problems – and this, of course excludes those who are dead. Table 1.3 shows the age standardised prevalence rate ratios, thus permitting more direct comparisons between groups. While the picture is not as clear cut as for mortality data, as discussed elsewhere[10], we see that on several measures the South Asian groups had more CHD than the general population, and nearly always more than the other ethnic groups, i.e., Chinese and African-Caribbean. It is worth noting that on the objective indicator of major Q waves on ECG, Indian men had substantially lower comparative prevalence than Pakistani and Bangladeshi men. This is important because the validity of self-reported data in multi-ethnic studies where languages and cultures differ is open to question.

For women the data were much less clear. Indian women reported both less angina and heart attack and had a lower comparative rate of Q waves on ECG. Self report data on Pakistani and Bangladeshi women were inconsistent, but Q waves on ECG

Table 1.2: Prevalence of IHD (heart attack or angina) or stroke by ethnic group (not age adjusted). Extracted from the Health Survey for England 1999[13].

	I	P	B	C	BC	G
Men -16 and over	8.2	4.8	5.1	2.9	4.8	8.5
Men - 55 and over	29.2	21.3	17.8	9.7	12.4	21.9
Women -16 and over	2.3	2.6	1.9	0.6	2.8	6.2
Women - 55 and over	10.1	16.8	6.3	2.5	8.9	15.5

Table 1.3: Directly standardised prevalence rate ratios for cardiovascular diseases (general population = 100) Extracted from the Health Survey for England 1999[13].

	I	P	B	C	BC
Men					
Angina - self	128	126	186	38	32
- RQ	170	79	139	26	97
Heart attack - self	95	144	168	32	14
- RQ (Possible MI)	85	77	140	41	88
E.C.G. - Major Q waves	86	147	178	60	68
Women					
Angina - self	95	126	109	20	111
- RQ	96	92	113	48	122
Heart attack - self	34	162	20	0	57
- RQ (possible MI)	99	155	182	59	115
E.C.G. major Q waves	84	92	20	65	66

I (Indian), P (Pakistani), B (Bangladeshi), C (Chinese), BC (Black Carribean), G (General population), RQ (Rose angina questionnaire), MI (myocardial infarction)

were comparatively less common, and in Bangladeshi women the ratio of 20% seems so low that it needs verification. The Newcastle Heart Project[12] only had 56 Bangladeshi women but none had probable CHD on ECG criteria, and the proportion with possible CHD on ECG criteria was, at 13%, lower than Indians, Pakistanis and Europeans.

As ethnic monitoring is not mandatory within primary care, there are currently little routine data available. However, data are available from the National Morbidity Statistics from General Practice study done in 1991[16]. Essentially 60 practices in England and Wales provided data for one year, on face-to-face contact with 502,493 patients. 2% of these patients were from ethnic minority groups compared to 6% in the 1991 census. Gill *et al* reported a re-analysis of the data[11]. This new analysis included consultations with a nurse (although the study did not record nurse consultations if a doctor was also consulted during the same visit). The standard population for calculating the standardised patient consulting ratios (SPCR) was the entire study population including those for whom there was no ethnicity code (17% of patients). Interpretation of the data requires caution as the sample was not representative, and the numbers of people was small.

In Indians, circulatory diseases were not one of the dominant presenting problems but the standardised ratio was comparatively high for endocrine disorders and circulatory conditions (ratio for all ages in men 135 and in women 117).

For Pakistanis the standardised ratio for the circulatory system was comparatively low (ratio 99 for men, 80 for women). There was a substantially raised standardised ratio for endocrine disorders. For Bangladeshis there was a high standardised ratio for endocrine diseases; and a huge difference in men (standardised ratio 144) and women (ratio 66) for circulatory disorders. The overall message from the morbidity data is of a substantial burden of disease, but with less excess in comparison to the population as a whole, than shown in mortality data[10, 11]. These findings also point to major differences between subgroups of the South Asian population and to differences between men and women. The low rates of CHD mortality in Bangladeshi women are echoed in the primary care morbidity data and in the prevalence of Q waves on ECG.

Hypotheses relating to ethnic variations and the excess in South Asians

The question of why South Asian populations are more susceptible to CHD will be explored from numerous perspectives. In general terms the explanations are:

1.   The high and excess mortality rates are statistical artefact. This is unlikely to be more than a partial explanation although it merits more attention than it has received.

2.   South Asians are more susceptible for genetic reasons.

3.   South Asians are more susceptible for non-genetic reasons, e.g., from metabolic adaptation in early life, then dysadaptation in later, middle age.

4.   The prevalence of classical causal factors is comparatively high in South Asians. This holds for insulin resistance and diabetes (all South Asian groups), smoking in Bangladeshi men, and lack of physical activity (all South Asian groups). It does not hold for smoking (in most South Asian groups), blood pressure and cholesterol.

5.   The prevalence of risk factors other than classical ones is high, e.g., Lp(a), homocysteine, infection, poverty, stress, etc.

6.   There is a potent interaction of known causal factors specific to South Asian groups.

7.   South Asians are less likely to die of other important causes, e.g., cancer, so a high rate of CHD is the consequence (the competing causes hypothesis). If the suggestion of a higher mortality without corresponding excesses in morbidity is corroborated, then this concept as well as difference in case fatality will need deeper study.

Many specific explanatory hypotheses have been generated but have not been studied with prospective research designs, in the required range of ethnic groups, in population settings and with sample sizes with sufficient power. Work thus far has generated numerous ideas including the effects of stress and racism, the use of ghee and other cooking oils, sub-clinical hypothyroidism, central obesity, insulin resistance, a thrifty genotype, a thrifty phenotype, low vitamin C, high homocysteine, endothelial dysfunction, differences in microalbuminuria, a greater burden of infection, high levels of Lp(a) and other specific lipid abnormalities. The possibility of varying susceptibility has been raised but a formal hypothesis has not been systematically studied. Rapid change in some risk factors may *per se* confer a risk beyond that predicted by a single measure e.g. Punjabis in Southall had a mean serum cholesterol of 6.5 mmol/l compared with 4.9 mmol/l for their siblings in Punjab,

India[17]. By inference, this reflects a rise after migration. Box 1.2 summarises many of the hypotheses discussed above.

Box 1.2: Some hypotheses to explain ethnic variations in cardiovascular disease

Hypothesis	Status
Variation in case fatality	Not studied but unlikely to be the full explanation.
Variation in prevalence of established classical risk factors	Rejected, mainly from cross-sectional data, with limited prospective studies. Needs fresh evaluation.
High prevalence of diabetes	Accepted as partial explanation.
Insulin resistance	Under rigorous test, with evidence of some limited explanatory value independent of diabetes
Hyperhomocysteinaemia	Supportive evidence from cross-sectional data
Psychosocial factors increasing stress	Not tested formally. Evidence of potential relevance from cross-sectional studies.
Socio-economic factors	Limited test in cross-sectional studies, but generally accepted not to fully explain ethnic group differences.
Racism	Not tested in the UK
Lp(a) excess	Under test in cross-sectional research
Chronic inflammation	Not tested, with limited data at cross-sectional level
Adaptation–dysadaptation hypothesis	Some evidence from India
Genetic factors, and gene-environment interactions	Not tested in a systematic way.
Access and quality of health care.	Not tested in a systematic way.
Varying effects of risk factors	Suggested but never tested in a formal way

One interesting explanation that has engaged attention is that South Asians have more insulin resistance, that is, they require larger amounts of the hormone insulin to maintain a normal blood sugar. This may be the result of different metabolism resulting from either genetic factors or environmental factors, or both. The fact that South Asians have more of their body fat on the trunk, rather than limbs, and such fat has different metabolic characteristics is possibly important here. These ideas are being explored intensively.

Another explanation which seems important is that adverse circumstances in the womb and early life increase the risk of a number of health problems, including CHD. The explanation offered is that metabolism is programmed in early life. If later there is a mismatch between the metabolism a person is programmed for and the lifestyle adopted, disease occurs. If the critical factor was a change in life circumstances, from that of the relatively poor, to that of the relatively wealthy, this explanation might apply to migrant groups who make that transition.

An overview of risk factors – the basis for prevention and control of CHD

While CHD mortality risk, to a large extent, is shared across South Asian subgroups, most risk factors vary enormously. Some data extracted from the HSE '99 is given in Table 1.4 and the text below also relates to the data in Gill *et al*'s health needs assessment [11]. Other papers in this monograph will deal with several of these risk factors in detail.

Indians are extremely heterogeneous, so findings are likely to differ in different places, and communities. In particular, religion has an important effect. For example, smoking is much less common in Sikhs than Hindus. The reverse applies to drinking alcohol. Indians have substantial needs in relation to smoking, alcohol and lack of physical activity. In women the cultural taboo against smoking is holding, for the present, but it is likely to relax in time with a consequent rise in the consumption of tobacco.

Vigorous action to control dyslipidaemia is warranted. Indians are relatively short and obesity (particularly central) is common. Indians born in the UK are growing

Table 1.4A: Pattern of key cardiovascular risk factors – prevalence means and age standardised ratios in men. Extracted from the Health Survey for England '99[13].

	I	P	B	C	BC	G
%current smoker	23	26	44	17	35	27
- Ratio	78	90	157	62	126	100
No physical activity (30 mins) in past 4 weeks	30	32	49	31	24	23
- Ratio of number of days	82	67	52	65	109	100
Blood pressure mean - systole	134	130	127	131	136	B137
-Ratio of mean systolic pressure	100	98	94	97	100	100
Obesity (BMI > 30kg/m^2)	12	13	5	6	18	19
- Ratio	66	74	32	38	102	100
LDL cholesterol (mean mmol/l)	3.5	3.2	3.3	3.4	3.30	3.5
- Ratio	100	91	94	95	98	100
HDL cholesterol (mmol/l)	1.3	1.1	1.1	1.3	1.5	1.3
- Ratio	99	87	83	101	114	100

Table 1.4B: Pattern of key cardiovascular risk factors – prevalence means and age standardised ratios in women. Extracted from the Health Survey for England '99[13].

	I	P	B	C	BC	G
% current smokers	6	5	1	9	25	27
- Ratio	19	14	7	31	85	1
No physical activity (30 mins) in past 4 weeks	35	39	54	31	25	28
- Ratio of number of days	71	62	37	72	105	100
Blood pressure mean - systole	126	123	120	125	129	133
- Ratio	99	102	97	98	101	100
Obesity (BMJ > 30kg/m^2)	102	161	63	20	160	100
LDL cholesterol (mean mmol/l)	3.1	3.0	-	2.9	3.1	3.5
- Ratio	99	89	-	94	95	100
HDL Cholesterol	1.4	1.4	1.3	1.6	1.6	1.6
- Ratio	92	88	88	99	103	100

I (Indian), P (Pakistani), B (Bangladeshi), C (Chinese), BC (Black Carribean), G (General population) taller than their parents. Blood pressures vary in different Indian communities, with the best judgement being that levels are similar to the white population, i.e. hypertension is a common disorder. Diabetes and the associated syndrome of insulin resistance are exceptionally common in men and women.

Pakistanis are mainly Muslims, whose religion impacts in ways important to health. Although heterogeneity between Pakistani communities should not be overlooked, this is less so than in Indians. As with Indians there are substantial needs in relation to smoking (men) and in promotion of physical activity. Few people drink alcohol, though the taboo against it may lead to underreporting. Those Pakistanis who do drink may have special difficulties due to social problems arising from admitting to an alcohol problem.

The comments above on lipids and physical measures of health including obesity in Indians, apply with even greater force in Pakistanis whose rates of heart disease and diabetes are slightly higher than in Indians. The reduction of cardiovascular and diabetes risk factors is the prime health need in Pakistani adults.

Of the South Asian populations in the UK the Bangladeshis are the most homogeneous, having in common a single major religion, Islam, and origins from a small country, Bangladesh, and within that many Bangladeshis come from Sylhet. Smoking prevalence in Bangladeshi men is exceptionally high, making this the priority public health issue. Although the prevalence of smoking is relatively low in Bangladeshi women tobacco chewing (with betel nut or paan) is a common practice, and much more so than in Indian or Pakistani women. The points made on alcohol use in Pakistanis apply to Bangladeshis too. The exceptionally low rates of physical activity (a major issue) need to be interpreted in the knowledge that most men are in manual occupations. Lipid patterns in Bangladeshis are problematic with the apparently low total cholesterol being a result of very low HDL cholesterol. This together with high triglycerides signifies a need for dietary advice and change.

Bangladeshis are very short, a reflection of poor nutrition in childhood. In comparison with other ethnic groups, Bangladeshis have less obesity and a lower mean blood pressure. This should not lead to complacency for their risk of developing cardiovascular disease and diabetes is the highest of all the ethnic groups considered here. It may be that cardiovascular risk is triggered at a lower threshold than in other ethnic groups.

Conclusions and recommendations

CHD is higher in South Asian groups than in the population as a whole, with increasing evidence that men in the poorest groups, of Pakistani and Bangladeshi origin, have the highest rates. The causes of the excess are incompletely understood. Recent work indicates that socio-economic factors are important. The role of the classic risk factors (high blood pressure, lipids, smoking) is vital. Central obesity and insulin resistance are two other factors of especial note.

The scale of the challenge, summarised in box 1.3, is too great for solitary and fragmented effort. The control of the CHD epidemic in South Asians requires a co-ordinated, vigorous response based on established principles and available evidence on effectiveness, and standards of care specified in guidelines such as the National Service Framework on CHD [18]. Practitioners must not await specific evidence from trials on South Asian populations (these are rare) or be deflected by scientific controversy. We should:

1.	Adopt broadly based strategies that focus on the established risk factors, take account of language and cultural needs, consider the issue of relative poverty (especially in Bangladeshis) and appreciate the heterogeneity of South Asians.

2.	Ensure that each of the known risk factors are vigorously tackled, including smoking cessation which has been relatively neglected. Smoking cessation services need to be targeted at Bangladeshi and Pakistani men, and at all South Asian teenagers. The other key risk factors requiring vigorous control include diabetes, hypertension, obesity, high fat diet, raised LDL cholesterol and lack of physical exercise. Disease registers and practice lists may need a valid ethnic code so services can be targeted.

3.	Use specific research in South Asians to help refine the above strategies. The main lesson to date is that practitioners should be particularly vigilant in controlling risk factors, for thresholds for intervention may be lower than in European origin populations (a topic for new research).

4.   Ensure that South Asian patients are well informed about CHD (there is evidence that their knowledge is low [19]). Community involvement will be needed to devise effective actions.

5.   Apply and audit agreed standards of care to achieve equity between ethnic groups in the quantity and quality of care.

Box 1.3: Challenges of ethnic variations in CHD

---

1.   Inclusion of the ethnic dimension without dividing society or creating racial disharmony.

2.   Creation of reliable information systems that provide information by ethnic, religious and language group.

3.   New and more stringent targets for disease control based on ethnic groups with the lowest rates of CHD.

4.   Value, learn from and utilise the heterogeneity of ethnic minority populations in both research and prevention.

5.   Seek understanding of differences in CHD frequency, i.e. hypothesis testing.

6.   Validate measurement methods for mortality, morbidity and risk factor data.

7.   Reduce disease (and risk factors prevalence), particularly in ethnic minority groups with high rates.

8.   In relation to preventive and therapeutic services avoid veering away from established paths, based on controlling the major classical risk factor, too readily.

9.   Achieve equity in service delivery, quality and outcome.

The South Asian community must be alerted to the epidemic and know the symptoms and signs of CHD so that early medical advice is sought. For South Asians, CHD will be a key health problem for many decades.

From the perspective of national and local Government and the National Health Service lost time needs to be made up. It seems incredible, looking back, that while attention focused on the "specific problems" of ethnic minority groups (e.g. birth control, weaning, rickets, surma, traditional medicines and macrocytic anaemia) an epidemic of cardiovascular disease was sweeping through the South Asian community, being the underlying cause of up to 50% of deaths. Why was this unnoticed? Why were there virtually no educational materials adapted or developed for ethnic minority groups until the last few years? These key questions reach to the core of the decision making process in research and health policy.

We need policies which offer equity in opportunity for escaping social and economic deprivation, and which give incentive to the NHS to meet both the mainstream and additional needs of ethnic minorities. The NHS needs to achieve the same levels of communication with, and quality of care for South Asians as it does for the general population. The achievement of such equity will require targeting of resources.

South Asians comprise one-quarter of the World's population. Globally, the epidemic in these populations threatens the international effort to bring the CHD epidemic to heel. South Asians comprise a substantial proportion of the population in most modern economies, particularly Britain. In Britain, South Asians are scattered throughout the country, so it is important that groups outside the London and Midlands areas are not overlooked.

Understanding cardiovascular diseases better will be of benefit nationally, not just to South Asians. Improving services to South Asians will, inevitably, raise standards for the whole population, and particularly other groups that are suffering from low quality or inequitable service. The work on CHD done in the U.K. will have global interest and value for CHD is poised to be the predominant killer in developing and industrialised countries alike.

The South Asian Health Foundation (SAHF), a new charity, has chosen a worthy challenge. SAHF has the potential to catalyse research in ethnic minorities and to foster high quality facilitation at educational events. SAHF's future symposia intend to involve a wider audience and reach out to all health care and allied professionals so that we can apply research from the cell to bedside to population.

Acknowledgements

I thank the many collaborators and co-investigators who have helped me gain understanding of the issues raised here. It is inevitably the case that one's own ideas can not be disentangled from those given by others. Sarah Wild has given permission for publication of Tables 1.1A and 1.1B for which I thank her. I have drawn upon work done with Paramjit Gill, Joe Kai and Sarah Wild in our joint Health Needs Assessment (ref. 11). I have also drawn on previous publications, sometimes written with others. I thank Hazel King for her secretarial support.

References

1. Adelstein A M. Some aspects of cardiovascular mortality in South Africa. Brit J Prev Soc Med 1963; 17:29-40.

2. Marmot M G, Adelstein A M, Bulusu L, Shukla V. Immigrant mortality in England and Wales 1970-78. (OPCS Studies on Population and Medical Subjects: No.47). London: HMSO, 1984.

3. Balarajan R. Ethnic differences in mortality from ischaemic heart disease and cerebrovascular disease in England and Wales. BMJ 1991;302:560-4.

4. Wild S, McKeigue P. Cross sectional analysis of mortality by country of birth in England and Wales, 1970-92. BMJ 1997;314:705-10.

5. Balarajan R. Ethnicity and variations in mortality from coronary heart disease. Health Trends 1996; 28: 45-51.

6. Harding S, Maxwell R. Differences in mortality of migrants. In Drever FWM, ed. Health Inequalities, pp 108-21. London: Office for National Statistics, 1997.

7. Nazroo JY. The Health of Britain's Ethnic Minorities. London: Policy Studies Institute, 1997.

8. Bhopal, R. S.; Hayes, L.: White, M.; Unwin, N.; Harland, J.; Ayis, S.; et al. Ethnic and socio-economic inequalities in coronary heart disease, diabetes and risk factors in Europeans and South Asians. Journal of Public Health Medicine. 2002; 24:95-105.

9. Gupta R, Gupta V P. Meta-analysis of coronary heart disease prevalence in India. Indian Heart Journal 1996;48:241.245.

10.   Bhopal R. What is the risk of coronary heart disease in South Asians? A review of UK research. Journal of Public Health Medicine 2000;22:375-385.

11.   Gill PS, Kai J, Bhopal RS, Wild S. Health Care Needs Assessment: Black and Minority Ethnic Groups. In: The epidemiologically based needs assessment reviews. Raftery J (ed). (Third Series.), 2002. (In press) available at: http://hcna.radcliffe-online.com/bemgframe.htm.

12.   Bhopal R, Unwin N, White M. et al. Heterogeneity of coronary heart disease risk factors in Indian, Pakistani, Bangladeshi and European origin populations: cross-sectional study. BMJ 1999; 319:215-20.

13.   Joint health services unit. Health Survey for England. The health of minority ethnic groups' 99. London, The stationery office, 2001.

14.   McKeigue P M, Marmot M G. Mortality from coronary heart disease in Asian communities in London. British Medical Journal 1988;297:903.

15.   Donaldson L J, Taylor J B. Patterns of Asian and Non-Asian morbidity in hospitals. British Medical Journal 1983; 286: 949-951.

16.   McCormick A, Fleming D, Charlton J. Morbidity Statistics from General Practice. Fourth national study 1991-1992. London: HMSO, 1995.

17.   Bhatnagar D, Anand, I S, Durrington P N et al. "Coronary risk factors in people from the Indian subcontinent living in west London and their siblings in India. Lancet 1995;345: 405-409.

18.   Department of Health. National Service Framework on Coronary Heart Disease. London, 2000.

19.   Rankin J, Bhopal R. Understanding of heart disease and diabetes in a South Asian community: cross sectional study testing the 'snowball' sample method. Pub Health 2001; 115: 253-260.

2

Conceptualising the causes of coronary heart disease in South Asians

J Kooner and J C Chambers

Epidemiology

As discussed by Bhopal in the previous chapter, the burden of cardiovascular disease is greatest amongst South Asians living in urban areas[1] and overseas compared to appropriate comparison populations[2-9]. South Asians represent the largest ethnic minority group in the UK. Amongst UK South Asians, mortality from coronary heart disease (CHD) is approximately 40% higher[2,3], and admission rates with myocardial infarction in one study were 2-fold higher[10] when compared with white Europeans. The increase in CHD risk is evident in each of the major South Asian subgroups[11,12] and is most striking in young males, amongst whom CHD mortality is at least 2-fold higher than in their white European counterparts[2].

Risk factors underlying CHD in South Asians

Diabetes and insulin resistance
Population studies have consistently identified a high prevalence of non-insulin dependent diabetes amongst urban and overseas South Asians. The prevalence of diabetes is reported as 2-5% in rural Indians, 5-10% in urban Indians, and almost 20% in UK South Asians, compared to 4% of white European males[13-21]. In the UK, South Asians develop diabetes on average 10 years earlier than their white European counterparts[22], and South Asians with diabetes show a markedly increased predisposition to cardiovascular disease. In a large prospective study, cardiovascular and CHD mortality were higher amongst South Asians with diabetes, compared with white Europeans[23]. Furthermore, circulatory disease accounted for 77% of deaths amongst

South Asians, compared with 46% amongst white Europeans[23]. In addition to the high prevalence of diabetes, insulin resistance and its related metabolic abnormalities (central obesity, glucose intolerance, elevated plasma insulin, increased triglycerides, raised PAI-1 (plasminogen activator inhibitor), and reduced HDL (high-density lipoprotein cholesterol)) are more common amongst South Asians than white Europeans populations (Table 2.1)[18,20,21,24]. It is estimated that diabetes and insulin resistance may account for up to 70% of major Q wave ECG abnormalities in UK South Asians[25].

Table 2.1. Coronary risk factors amongst UK South Asian and white European males in West London (adapted from ref. 18).

	White Europeans	UK South Asians			
		Punjabi Sikh	Punjabi Hindu	Gujarati Hindu	Muslim
Cigarette smoking (%)	30	4	21	33	30
Systolic BP (mmHg)	121	128	126	122	120
Total cholesterol (mmol/L)	6.1	6.1	5.9	5.5	6.0
Diabetes (%)	5	20	19	22	19
Waist-hip ratio	0.93	0.98	0.98	0.98	0.97
2hr insulin (mU/L)	19	39	42	49	43
Fasting triglycerides (mmol/L)	1.48	1.73	1.74	1.49	1.85
HDL cholesterol (mmol/L)	1.24	1.22	1.17	1.14	1.04

The mechanisms underlying the relationship between insulin resistance and CHD remain to be determined. Hyperglycaemia, hyperinsulinaemia, dyslipidaemia, a prothrombotic state, and hypertension may each have a separate contribution[26-28]. Elevated fasting and post-glucose load glucose concentrations are associated with increased risk of CHD, even in subjects without diabetes[29-31]. Hyperglycaemia may contribute to accelerated atherosclerosis through glycation of collagen and lipoproteins, generation of reactive oxygen species, and impaired vascular endothelial function, as discussed by Shah and Kearney in chapter 4[32-34]. Hyperinsulinaemia may promote atherosclerosis through increasing blood pressure, smooth muscle cell proliferation, release of PAI-1, and inhibition of fibrinolysis[27,35,36]. However, the beneficial effects of insulin therapy on risk of CHD events in patients with type 2 diabetes argue against hyperinsulinaemia as the primary atherogenic defect in insulin resistant states. A reduction in insulin mediated adipocyte lipogenesis secondary to insulin resistance may be of more importance[28,.37]. Insulin resistance is associated with increased levels of free fatty acids, which leads to an increase in hepatic VLDL synthesis, hypertriglyceridaemia, a reduction in HDL cholesterol and an increase in atherogenic small dense LDL[28,38]. This pattern of dyslipidaemia is associated with increased entry of cholesterol into, and reduced clearance of cholesterol from, the arterial wall. Observations that CHD mortality is low in Afro-caribbeans[3,39] who have a high prevalence of insulin resistance and hypertension, but a favourable lipoprotein profile[40,41], suggest that the dyslipidaemia associated with insulin resistance may underlie CHD. However, the validity of this view is open to debate and discussed in later chapters.

Conventional CHD risk factors

High CHD mortality is shared by Hindu, Sikh and Muslim Asians[11,12]. In contrast, population studies have shown that levels of cigarette smoking, blood pressure and cholesterol, are not consistently raised in all South Asian groups (Table 2.1). These findings have led to the belief that conventional risk factors alone do not contribute to high CHD mortality rates in Asians despite making an important contribution[18].

The importance of conventional risk factors underlying increased CHD risk in urban, and overseas South Asians is further illustrated by comparisons of risk factors between migrant, and non-migrant Asians. Serum cholesterol, blood pressure, smoking rates, and BMI are all substantially higher in urban compared to rural Indians[42-46]. Similar differences exist amongst overseas South Asians compared to their non-migrant siblings[47] (Table 2.2). These observations support the view that classic risk factors impact on the high CHD rates in urban, and overseas South Asians, although the precise extent to which each contributes to increased CHD risk in Asians remains to be determined.

Other risk factors for CHD

A key question is whether diabetes, insulin resistance and the established CHD risk factors account for the increased risk of CHD amongst South Asians, compared to other populations. To date, no large scale prospective study has examined CHD mortality in South Asians, or its relationship to CHD risk factors. Much of the evidence is based upon the results of cross-sectional studies, which have compared risk factors between South Asians and other population groups. In West London, there was a 1.4-fold excess of pathological Q waves, a surrogate marker of CHD, amongst South Asians compared to Europeans[25]. After adjustment for age, smoking, cholesterol, fasting and 2 hour insulin, waist-hip ratio and glucose intolerance, there remained a 1.5-fold excess of pathological Q waves amongst South Asians. Similarly in Canada, South Asian ethnicity is associated with an excess of prevalent CHD, that is not accounted for by conventional risk factors, diabetes, HDL cholesterol, PAI-1 or fibrinogen[24]. The results of these studies suggest that other risk factors contribute to the observed excess CHD mortality amongst South Asians.

a) Inflammation and CHD in South Asians

Inflammation, as discussed later by Gupta in chapter 7, is now widely recognized as a central feature of atherogenesis, and in particular seems to play a critical role in destabilization of the fibrous cap tissue, predisposing to plaque rupture[48]. C-reactive protein (CRP), the classical acute phase reactant, is an extremely sensitive systemic marker of inflammation.

Recent studies indicate that CRP concentrations are higher in healthy asymptomatic South Asians, than in white Europeans[49]. In both populations CRP concentrations are closely associated with central obesity, and markers of insulin resistance (Figure 2.1). This is consistent with experimental studies which suggest that abdominal adipose tissue is a major source of cytokines, including IL-6, an important determinant of hepatic CRP synthesis[50,51]. The difference in CRP concentrations between South Asians and Europeans may be accounted for by the higher level of central obesity and insulin resistance in Asians[49]. These observations suggest that inflammatory activity is increased amongst South Asian, and white European subjects with the insulin resistance syndrome, and raise the possibility that inflammatory mechanisms underlie part of the increased risk of CHD, amongst insulin resistant South Asians.

Table 2.2. Coronary risk factors amongst UK South Asian men in West London, and their non-migrant male siblings in India (adapted from ref. 47). (NS=non significant)

	West London	Punjab	P=
Age (years)	46.0 ± 10.6	44.4 ± 9.4	NS
Body mass index (kg/m^2)	26.8 ± 5.2	22.9 ± 4.7	<0.001
Systolic BP (mmHg)	146 ± 23	132 ± 22	<0.001
Diastolic BP (mmHg)	93 ± 14	87 ± 12	<0.001
Total cholesterol (mmol/L)	6.5 ± 1.4	4.9 ± 1.1	<0.001
HDL cholesterol (mmol/L)	1.12 ± 0.45	1.21 ± 0.43	NS
Triglycerides (mmol/L)	2.10 (1.88-2.35)	2.06 (1.78-2.38)	NS
Fasting glucose (mmol/L)	5.7 ± 1.4	4.5 ± 1.0	<0.001
Fasting insulin (mU/L)	8.4 (7.2-9.8)	6.7 (5.4-8.4)	NS

Figure 2.1: Comparison of CRP concentrations between healthy asymptomatic South Asians and white Europeans

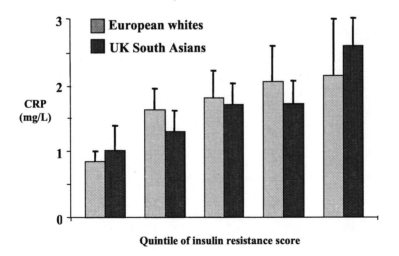

b) Endothelial dysfunction and CHD in South Asians

Endothelium dependent dilatation is impaired in healthy UK South Asians compared to white Europeans and is discussed further by Shah and Kearney in chapter 4.

c) Homocysteine and risk of CHD in South Asians

Recent studies show that concentrations of plasma homocysteine, an emerging risk factor for CHD, are higher in South Asians than white Europeans[20,24,52], suggesting that elevated homocysteine may contribute to increased CHD mortality in South Asians. Amongst South Asians, elevated homocysteine is accounted for by reduced concentrations of vitamins B_{12} and folate, compared to white Europeans[20]. In contrast, the MTHFR C677T mutation, identified as a major determinant of homocysteine concentrations in Europeans, is less prevalent and does not influence homocysteine concentrations in South Asians[53]. Whether the increased CHD risk in this group can be reduced by dietary supplementation with homocysteine-lowering B vitamins[54], remains to be determined.

d) Lipoprotein (a)

Lipoprotein (a), formed from the assembly of the protein apolipoprotein (a), has been identified as an independent risk factor for vascular disease, including CHD[55-57]. The mechanisms underlying this relationship is uncertain, but *in vitro* studies suggest that lipoprotein (a) may influence cholesterol uptake, and inhibit fibrinolysis[55]. Serum lipoprotein (a) concentrations are influenced primarily by genetic factors[58], with over 30 apolipoprotein (a) alleles identified to date[59]. Lipoprotein (a) concentrations are reported to be higher in South Asians compared to white Europeans, and Chinese, and may influence CHD risk in this group[24,47,60].

e) Low birth weight

South Asian babies are small compared to other populations. The average weight of a newborn native Indian is 2.7kg, compared with 3.1kg in UK South Asians, 3.2kg in Chinese and Afro-caribbeans, 3.4kg in Caucasians, and 3.7kg in North American Indians (Table 2.3)[61-66]. The possibility that low-birth weight may contribute to increased risk of CHD amongst South Asians is supported by observations that the prevalence of CHD is significantly higher amongst Indians with birthweight <2.5kg, compared a birth-weight >3.2kg. This is discussed further by Fall in chapter 5.

f) Socio-economic factors

South Asians are more likely to live in areas with increased social and economic deprivation[67]. In addition, the results of several studies provide evidence that UK South Asians have different access to health care. Although South Asians are more likely than Europeans to seek medical advice for symptoms suggestive of angina[68], regional studies suggest that South Asians may be less likely to be referred for exercise testing, wait longer to be seen by a cardiologist, wait longer for angiography, and be less likely to receive thrombolysis for acute myocardial infarction[69-72]. The contribution of socio-economic deprivation, and reduced provision of healthcare services, to increased CHD mortality needs wider investigation and is discussed further in chapter 12 by Williams and Harding.

Table 2.3. Mean birth weight, and incidence of low birth weight (<2500g), amongst different Ethnic groups in the UK (adapted from ref. 62)

	Mean Birthweight (g)	Incidence of low birth weight (%)
South Asian	3082 ± 527	10.1
Afro-Caribbean	3156 ± 604	9.4
African	3214 ± 617	9.2
Oriental	3231 ± 532	6.6
White European	3377 ± 548	5.0

Mechanisms underlying diabetes and insulin resistance in South Asians

Many accept the notion that diabetes and insulin resistance are major determinants of the increased CHD mortality amongst UK South Asians. Reasons underlying the higher prevalence of insulin resistance in UK South Asians are not known. Studies in white Europeans indicate that diabetes and insulin resistance may be influenced by genetic and environmental factors, the latter include reduced physical activity, increased weight, and dietary intake.

Environmental factors

UK South Asians have higher glucose and insulin concentrations, an increased prevalence of diabetes, and lower HDL cholesterol, compared to non-migrant Asians (Table 2.2)[47]. These observations demonstrate that environmental factors may contribute to insulin resistance in UK South Asians.

1. Obesity

Amongst Europeans, obesity, and in particular visceral adiposity, is associated with reduced insulin sensitivity, and an increased risk of diabetes and CHD[73]. Population studies have shown that UK South Asians (except Bangladeshis) have similar BMIs, to white Europeans[18,20,24,74,75]. Although this might suggest that adiposity does not account for insulin resistance amongst South Asians, this comparison may be misleading, since South Asians have greater visceral adiposity than white Europeans, for the same level of BMI[18,74,75]. Previous studies show that visceral adiposity is closely associated with insulin resistance and its related metabolic disturbances, diabetes, inflammation, and CHD, amongst South Asians[18,25,49,74-76]. The reasons underlying the disproportionate increase in visceral adiposity amongst UK South Asians are not known.

2. Dietary factors

Diet plays an important role in the development of insulin resistance. In North American and white European populations, a diet high in saturated fatty acids is associated with obesity, hyperglycaemia and hyperinsulinaemia[77-79] and an increased risk of diabetes and CHD[79-85]. In addition, trans fatty acids (TFA), primarily derived from commercial hydrogenation of polyunsaturated oils[86] have been associated with raised triglycerides, and raised total to HDL cholesterol ratio, and an increase in post-prandial hyperinsulinaemia, suggesting an effect of TFA on insulin sensitivity[87,88]. Diet may also have protective factors. Starchy foods producing relatively flat glycaemic responses, are associated with weight loss, reduced blood pressure, and lower glucose, insulin, and lipid levels[89,90]. Phytoestrogens such as genestein and daidzen, may also confer protection from atherosclerosis, through an action on the oestrogen receptor. Phytoestrogens raise HDL cholesterol, and lower total cholesterol and total / HDL cholesterol ratio, and may improve insulin sensitivity[91,92].

The dietary mechanisms underlying the increased prevalence of insulin resistance, and related metabolic disturbances, amongst UK South Asians are not known. Studies based upon weighed 7 day food diaries, have reported that UK South Asians have higher intakes of polyunsaturated fat, and carbohydrate, and lower total and saturated fat intakes, compared to White Europeans (Table 2.4)[93]. In this study, insulin levels were closely correlated with total and saturated fat intake in Europeans only, suggesting that dietary fat may contribute to reduced insulin sensitivity in Europeans, but not Asians. These observations have lead some to describe the diet of UK South Asians as favourable and to propose that increased insulin resistance in South Asians is largely determined by genetic factors.

Table 2.4. Dietary intake amongst rural South Asians, UK South Asians, and white Europeans (adapted from refs. 93 and 94).

	South Asians			European whites
	Rural S Asia	Urban UK	UK	
Energy (MJ/day)	9.2	8.9	9.5	10.8
Fat (% of energy intake)	15	25	37	39
Polyunsaturate / saturate ratio	0.66	0.62	0.50	0.40
Carbohydrates (% of energy intake)	73	62	46	41
Protein (% energy)	12	13	14	15
Fibre (g/day)	24	25	29	18

However, there are important limitations in our understanding of the relationship between environmental factors and insulin resistance in UK South Asians. The relationship of dietary intake with concentrations of HDL cholesterol, triglycerides, and glucose (key components of the metabolic syndrome), or with other conventional CHD risk factors, has not been investigated. Similarly, there is a paucity of data on the intake of TFAs, high-glycaemic foods, and of phyto-oestrogens in South Asians (as reviewed by Sanders in chapter 9). Furthermore, studies based on 7 day food diaries have important limitations. Food diaries rely upon accurate knowledge of the nutritional content of individual foodstuffs. Whilst some of this information is available from sources such as the UK Food Tables, nutrient content is not available for many European dishes, and is limited for many South Asian foods.

Comparisons between Europeans and South Asians, also do not address the changes in insulin sensitivity that have occurred with migration from India. Indeed, no study has examined the dietary changes that have occurred with migration, and their possible contribution to insulin sensitivity amongst UK South Asians. Observations that total fat constitutes less than 15% of energy in rural India, compared with over 30% in the UK (Table 4.4)[94], suggest that increased total or saturated fat intake may contribute to reduced insulin sensitivity in UK South Asians. Careful studies of the differences in dietary habit between UK and non-migrant South Asians, are needed to define the role of diet in determining CHD amongst UK South Asians.

3. Physical activity

Physical inactivity is recognised as a risk factor for diabetes, obesity, CHD, and cardiovascular mortality in North American and white European populations[95-98]. In prospective studies, physical inactivity increases risk of CHD by up to two-fold, comparable to the risk associated with conventional CHD risk factors such as cigarette smoking and hypertension. Increasing evidence suggests that the adverse effects of physical inactivity on CHD risk. may be mediated by insulin resistance. An increase in physical activity is associated with a reduction in weight, serum insulin, hyperuricaemia, diastolic blood pressure, and increased HDL cholesterol[99]. Increased physical activity may also prevent the onset of diabetes[100]. White, in chapter 12, discusses further physical inactivity in South Asians as a risk factor for CHD.

4. Genetic factors

Family studies, in other populations, have shown that a component of insulin resistance is inherited[101]. In Mexican Americans, insulin resistance segregates as a familial trait and evidence for linkage has been found between chromosome 6q and insulin action[102]. This chromosomal region contains the gene for a protein which may be an inhibitor of insulin-receptor tyrosine kinase[103,104]. In white type 2 diabetic pedigrees, segregation analysis suggests the presence of a major autosomal locus determining 33% of the variance in fasting insulin[105]. Support for the hypothesis that a component of insulin resistance is inherited in South Asians, comes from observations of hyperinsulinaemia and impaired NEFA suppression, after an oral glucose load, in non-diabetic first degree relatives of UK South Asian survivors of premature MI (Figure 2.2)[106]. In recent studies, an increase in central and generalised adiposity, both closely associated with insulin sensitivity in cross-sectional studies, have been linked to the –55 C-T mutations of the mitochondrial uncoupling protein UCP3[107]. However, the mutation is associated with obesity in females only, and there is no increased prevalence of the mutation amongst South Asians compared to Europeans. The genetic factors underlying reduced insulin sensitivity and increased CHD amongst South Asians remain to be determined and is further discussed by Samani and Sharma in chapter 6.

Figure 2.2: Observations of hyperinsulinaemia and impaired NEFA suppression, after an oral glucose load, in non-diabetic first degree relatives of UK South Asian survivors of premature MI (PSMI=survivors of premature MI, PMC=control subjects).

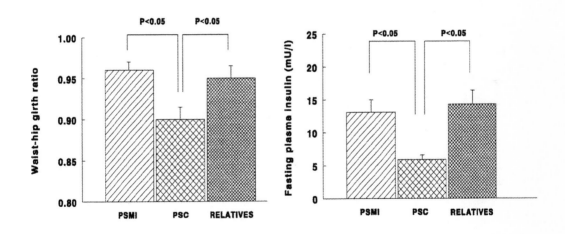

Management of CHD risk factors in UK South Asians

CHD has a multifactorial aetiology, and coronary risk factors have a multiplicative effect. Effective prevention therefore requires identification and treatment of the total burden of risk, rather than single risk factors.

Diabetes and Insulin resistance

Cardiovascular disease is the principal cause of death amongst patients with diabetes[23]. The prevalence of diabetes is four-fold higher in South Asians than Europeans[18-20], and diabetes is present in over 50% of South Asian CHD patients[20]. Diabetes is therefore of particular importance in this ethnic group. The results of recent studies amongst white Europeans provide unequivocal evidence that in patients with diabetes, the incidence of myocardial infarction can be reduced by 21% through rigorous blood pressure control (target: <130/80 mmHg), and by 16% through tight control of blood glucose (target: fasting plasma glucose <6.0 mmol/L)[108,109]. Achieving these targets should be a priority in the management, and prevention, of CHD in UK South Asians.

A major limitation in the treatment of insulin resistance, is the lack of solid evidence that improved insulin sensitivity is associated with a reduction in CHD mortality. Nevertheless, weight reduction, and increased physical activity are accepted measures to improve insulin sensitivity[110,111], and may prevent the onset of diabetes[100]. In the future, novel insulin sensitising agents, such as the thiazolidinediones, may have important consequences in South Asians[112,113]. Weight loss can be achieved merely by reducing the fat content of the diet without the need to voluntarily restrict food intake[114]. In UK South Asians, energy intake from fat is twice that of non-migrants[115,116]. The most important practical measure is reducing the quantity of fat/oil used in preparation of foods. Most South Asians live in extended family units, and food is generally prepared at home. Targeted education of the 'shopper and cook' can be highly effective, and thus have a significant impact on the diet of other high-risk members of the family. Physical activity levels in Asians are low. Moderate activity including walking, swimming, cycling will have energy expenditures of about 100 kcal/h, and should be undertaken daily. It is important to maintain increased physical activity, otherwise the effects on insulin resistance are short lived.

Conventional risk factors

As discussed by Bhopal in chapter 1, cigarette smoking rates are higher in Bangladeshi men, and similar in muslim men, compared to white Europeans. Cigarette smoking is one of the most important predictors of MI in South Asians[117]. For individuals currently smoking 10 or more per day the odds ratio for CHD is raised substantially. Often, success on smoking cessation is greatest after the acute event. Smoking cessation may reduce CHD by about 25% in South Asian men. South Asian women have very low smoking rates. Health promotion such as that discussed by Zaidi in chapter 10, aims to ensure that smoking rates should not rise in second generation UK South Asians.

Primary and secondary prevention studies show that cholesterol lowering reduces CHD risk, even amongst subjects with average cholesterol levels[142-144]. In this regard, 'normal' cholesterol levels, often based on a range between 4.0-6.5 mmol/l, should be re-defined. Total cholesterol levels have risen by almost 2mmol/L with migration to the UK from India[47] and undoubtedly have a major influence on the high CHD rates in UK South Asians. Drug therapy to lower cholesterol should be considered in all high-risk South Asians, irrespective of baseline cholesterol level[118]. Many South Asians have high triglycerides and low HDL cholesterol, and increased small dense LDL cholesterol[18,20,24,25]. The data from clinical and metabolic studies linking mild to moderate hypertriglyceridaemia and low HDL cholesterol to CHD is compelling[119-121] and would favour treatment of this atherogenic phenotype. Ideally, in UK South Asians, the lipid profile should be similar to non-migrants; total cholesterol should not exceed 4.5 mmol/, LDL cholesterol 2.5 mmol/l, triglycerides 1.5 mmol/l, and HDL cholesterol should be higher than 1.0mmol/l. These values are acceptable because they are similar to rural populations at low risk of CHD[47].

Hypertension in South Asians is discussed by Agyemang and Bhopal in chapter 8. Undoubtedly, raised blood pressure is a strong predictor of CHD[122], and randomised trials indicate that antihypertensive therapy is effective in reducing CHD and stroke rates[123,124]. Active attempts should be made to detect, and control hypertension in South Asian subjects. In middle aged UK South Asians, blood pressure levels should probably not exceed the non-migrant blood pressure of 140/85 mmHg in men and women[47].

Identification of South Asians at increased CHD risk

Therapeutic intervention to reduce CHD events should be directed to patients with proven CHD; first degree relatives of patients with premature CHD; and to individuals who are asymptomatic, but at high risk of CHD. To identify these high-risk persons, the American College of Cardiology, the American Heart Association, and the European

Society of Cardiology, have recommended adoption of the Framingham CHD risk assessment equations[125-128]. The Framingham equations predict CHD risk accurately amongst predominantly white populations in North America, and Europe[129-132]. However, the validity of extrapolating risk functions to populations other than those from which they were derived, remains to be established[133].

In recent studies we have evaluated the validity of the Framingham functions amongst UK South Asians[134]. We found that CHD mortality rates were almost 2-fold higher amongst South Asian, than white European males. In contrast, the CHD mortality rate predicted by the Framingham functions amongst a representative sample of UK South Asians, is no different to the predicted rate in Europeans. The Framingham functions therefore underestimate the risk of CHD amongst South Asians by approximately 50% (Figure 2.3)[134]. This may reflect the failure of these functions to take account of insulin resistance and related disturbances. A logical solution to this problem might be to lower the threshold for treatment in UK South Asians, although the validity of this approach remains to be determined.

Identification of South Asians at increased CHD risk therefore presents a major obstacle for the clinician. Most studies support the view that insulin resistance is the key disturbance underlying increased CHD risk in UK South Asians. However, the absence of a simple, reproducible marker of insulin resistance presents a further problem to the clinician. In practice, the combination of raised fasting triglycerides (>1.5 mmol/l), low HDL cholesterol (<1.0 mmol/l), raised fasting glucose (>6.0mmol/l), central obesity (waist-hip girth ratio >1.0 in men, and >0.85 in women), and hypertension, reliably identifies insulin resistant subjects, who are likely to benefit most from risk factor modification.

Conclusions and future directions

Future work is necessary to identify the precise environmental and genetic mechanisms underlying insulin resistance and increased CHD risk in UK South Asians. Identification of dietary factors, and nutrient-gene interactions, underlying insulin resistance, and increased risk of CHD, amongst South Asians will enable formulation of novel strategies for dietary intervention for CHD in Asians.

Investigation of the heritability of metabolic disturbances within large, extended South Asian families, may provide important insights into genetic factors determining CHD risk. Large-scale association studies and ultimately whole genome association studies to discover patterns of genetic variation leading to insulin resistance and atherosclerotic CVD in the South Asians should provide key insights into metabolic pathways involved and disease pathogenesis.

Figure 2.3: CHD risk prediction and observed rates of CHD in UK South Asians and white Europeans.

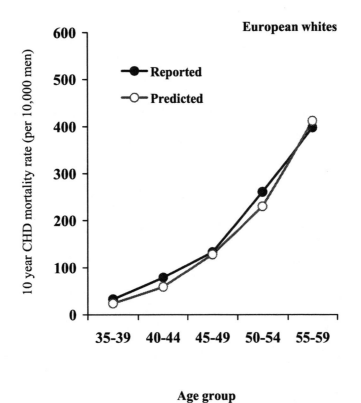

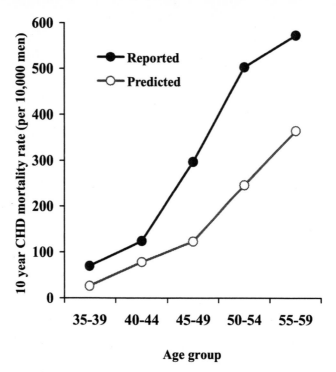

UK South Asians

Age group

The identification of disease-associated genes will have broad implications for management of these disorders in all ethnic groups. The failure of the Framingham risk functions to predict increased CHD risk in UK South Asians, also demonstrates the need for prospective population studies in South Asians, to enable the development of strategies, and risk prediction models, that identify South Asians at increased CHD risk. Finally, novel treatment strategies are needed for subjects with insulin resistance, and controlled clinical trials are necessary to assess the effectiveness of treatment, specifically in this ethnic group.

References

1.   Chadha SL, Gopinath N, Shekhawat S. Urban-rural differences in the prevalence of coronary heart disease and its risk factors in Delhi. Bull World Health Organ 1997; 75:31-38.

2.   Balarajan R. Ethnicity and variations in mortality from coronary heart disease. Health Trends 1996; 28:45-51.

3. Wild S, McKeigue P. Cross sectional analysis of mortality by country of birth in England and Wales, 1970-92. BMJ 1997; 314:705-710.

4. Sheth T, Nair C, Nargundkar M, Anand S, Yusuf S. Cardiovascular and cancer mortality among Canadians of European, south Asian and Chinese origin from 1979 to 1993: an analysis of 1.2 million deaths. CMAJ 1999; 161:132-138.

5. Chen AJ. Recent trends in the mortality and morbidity of cardiovascular diseases. Ann Acad Med Singapore 1980; 9:411-415.

6. Seedat YK. The prevalence of hypertension and the status of cardiovascular health in South Africa. Ethn Dis 1998; 8:394-397.

7. Miller GJ, Beckles GL, Maude GH, Carson DC, Alexis SD, Price SG, Byam NT. Ethnicity and other characteristics predictive of coronary heart disease in a developing community: principal results of the St James Survey, Trinidad. Int J Epidemiol 1989; 18:808-817.

8. Collins VR, Dowse GK, Cabealawa S, Ram P, Zimmet PZ. High mortality from cardiovascular disease and analysis of risk factors in Indian and Melanesian Fijians. Int J Epidemiol 1996; 25:59-69.

9. McKeigue PM, Miller GJ, Marmot MG. Coronary heart disease in south Asians overseas: a review. J Clin Epidemiol 1989; 42:597-609.

10. Wilkinson P, Sayer J, Laji K, Grundy C, Marchant B, Kopelman P, Timmis AD. Comparison of case fatality in south Asian and white patients after acute myocardial infarction: observational study. BMJ 1996; 312:1330-1333.

11. Balarajan R, Bulusu L, Adelstein AM, Shukla V. Patterns of mortality among migrants to England and Wales from the Indian subcontinent. BMJ 1984; 289:1185-1187.

12. Balarajan R, Raleigh VS. Patterns of mortality among Bangladeshis in England and Wales. Ethn Health 1997; 2:5-12.

13. Ramachandran A, Snehalatha C, Latha E, Manoharan M, Vijay V. Impacts of urbanisation on the lifestyle and on the prevalence of diabetes in native Asian Indian population. Diabetes Res Clin Pract 1999; 44:207-213.

14. Patandin S, Bots ML, Abel R, Valkenburg HA. Impaired glucose tolerance and diabetes mellitus in a rural population in south India. Diabetes Res Clin Pract 1994; 24:47-53.

15.   Wander GS, Khurana SB, Gulati R, Sachar RK, Gupta RK, Khurana S, Anand IS. Epidemiology of coronary heart disease in a rural Punjab population-- prevalence and correlation with various risk factors. Indian Heart J 1994; 46:319-323.

16.   Ramachandran A, Snehalatha C, Shyamala P, Vijay V, Viswanathan M. High prevalence of NIDDM and IGT in an elderly south Indian population with low rates of obesity. Diabetes Care 1994; 17:1190-1192.

17.   Singh RB, Bajaj S, Niaz MA, Rastogi SS, Moshiri M. Prevalence of type 2 diabetes mellitus and risk of hypertension and coronary artery disease in rural and urban population with low rates of obesity. Int J Cardiol 1998; 66:65-72.

18.   McKeigue PM, Shah B, Marmot MG. Relation of central obesity and insulin resistance with high diabetes prevalence and cardiovascular risk in South Asians. Lancet 1991; 337:382-386.

19.   Mather HM, Keen H. The Southall Diabetes Survey: prevalence of known diabetes in Asians and Europeans. BMJ 1985; 291:1081-1084.

20.   Chambers JC, Obeid OA, Refsum H, Ueland P, Hackett D, Hooper J, Turner RM, Thompson SG, Kooner JS. Plasma homocysteine concentrations and risk of coronary heart disease in UK South Asian and European men. Lancet 2000; 355:523-527.

21.   Bhopal R, Unwin N, White M, Yallop J, Walker L, Alberti KG, Harland J, Patel S, Ahmad N, Turner C, Watson B, Kaur D, Kulkarni A, Laker M, Tavridou A. Heterogeneity of coronary heart disease risk factors in Indian, Pakistani, Bangladeshi, and European origin populations: cross sectional study. BMJ 1999; 319:215-220.

22.   Nicholl CG, Levy JC, Mohan V, Rao PV, Mather HM. Asian diabetes in Britain: a clinical profile. Diabet Med 1986; 3:257-260.

23.   Mather HM, Chaturvedi N, Fuller JH. Mortality and morbidity from diabetes in South Asians and Europeans: 11-year follow-up of the Southall Diabetes Survey, London, UK. Diabet Med 1998; 15:53-59.

24.   Anand SS, Yusuf S, Vuksan V, Devanesen S, Teo KK, Montague PA, Kelemen L, Yi C, Lonn E, Gerstein H, Hegele RA, McQueen M. Differences in risk factors, atherosclerosis, and cardiovascular disease between ethnic groups in Canada: the Study of Health Assessment and Risk in Ethnic groups (SHARE). Lancet 2000; 356:279-284.

25. McKeigue PM, Ferrie JE, Pierpoint T, Marmot MG. Association of early-onset coronary heart disease in South Asian men with glucose intolerance and hyperinsulinemia. Circulation 1993; 87:152-161.

26. Nathan DM, Meigs J, Singer DE. The epidemiology of cardiovascular disease in type 2 diabetes mellitus: how sweet it is ... or is it? Lancet 1997; 350 Suppl 1:SI4-9.

27. Yudkin JS. Abnormalities of coagulation and fibrinolysis in insulin resistance. Evidence for a common antecedent? Diabetes Care 1999; 22 Suppl 3:C25-30.

28. Ginsberg HN. Insulin resistance and cardiovascular disease. J Clin Invest 2000; 106:453-458.

29. Gerstein HC, Pais P, Pogue J, Yusuf S. Relationship of glucose and insulin levels to the risk of myocardial infarction: a case-control study. J Am Coll Cardiol 1999; 33:612-619.

30. Balkau B, Bertrais S, Ducimetiere P, Eschwege E. Is there a glycemic threshold for mortality risk? Diabetes Care 1999; 22:696-699.

31. Rodriguez BL, Lau N, Burchfiel CM, Abbott RD, Sharp DS, Yano K, Curb JD. Glucose intolerance and 23-year risk of coronary heart disease and total mortality: the Honolulu Heart Program. Diabetes Care 1999; 22:1262-1265.

32. Mohanty P, Hamouda W, Garg R, Aljada A, Ghanim H, Dandona P. Glucose challenge stimulates reactive oxygen species (ROS) generation by leucocytes. J Clin Endocrinol Metab 2000; 85:2970-2973.

33. Ho FM, Liu SH, Liau CS, Huang PJ, Lin-Shiau SY. High glucose-induced apoptosis in human endothelial cells is mediated by sequential activations of c-Jun NH(2)-terminal kinase and caspase-3. Circulation 2000; 101:2618-2624.

34. Williams SB, Goldfine AB, Timimi FK, Ting HH, Roddy MA, Simonson DC, Creager MA. Acute hyperglycemia attenuates endothelium-dependent vasodilation in humans in vivo. Circulation 1998; 97:1695-1701.

35. Meigs JB, Mittleman MA, Nathan DM, Tofler GH, Singer DE, Murphy-Sheehy PM, Lipinska I, D'Agostino RB, Wilson PW. Hyperinsulinemia, hyperglycemia, and impaired hemostasis: the Framingham Offspring Study. JAMA 2000; 283:221-228.

36. Festa A, D'Agostino R, Mykkanen L, Tracy RP, Zaccaro DJ, Hales CN, Haffner SM. Relative contribution of insulin and its precursors to fibrinogen and PAI-1 in a large population with different states of glucose tolerance. The Insulin Resistance Atherosclerosis Study (IRAS). Arterioscler Thromb Vasc Biol 1999; 19:562-568.

37. Verges BL. Dyslipidaemia in diabetes mellitus. Review of the main lipoprotein abnormalities and their consequences on the development of atherogenesis. Diabetes Metab 1999; 25 Suppl 3:32-40.

38. Grundy SM. Hypertriglyceridemia, atherogenic dyslipidemia, and the metabolic syndrome. Am J Cardiol 1998; 81:18B-25B.

39. Balarajan R. Ethnic differences in mortality from ischaemic heart disease and cerebrovascular disease in England and Wales. BMJ 1991; 302:560-564.

40. Zoratti R, Godsland IF, Chaturvedi N, Crook D, Crook D, Stevenson JC, McKeigue PM. Relation of plasma lipids to insulin resistance, nonesterified fatty acid levels, and body fat in men from three ethnic groups: relevance to variation in risk of diabetes and coronary disease. Metabolism 2000; 49:245-252.

41. Chaturvedi N, McKeigue PM, Marmot MG. Relationship of glucose intolerance to coronary risk in Afro-Caribbeans compared with Europeans. Diabetologia 1994; 37:765-772.

42. Singh RB, Rastogi V, Niaz MA, Ghosh S, Sy RG, Janus ED. Serum cholesterol and coronary artery disease in populations with low cholesterol levels: the Indian paradox. Int J Cardiol 1998; 65:81-90.

43. Reddy KK, Ramachandraiah T, Reddanna P, Thyagaraju K. Serum lipid peroxides and lipids in urban and rural Indian men. Arch Environ Health 1994; 49:123-127.

44. Swaroop V, Agnihotri MS. Smoking habits, its forms and impact on pulmonary health in planes of Uttar Pradesh. J Indian Med Assoc 1998; 96:80-81.

45. Singh RB, Sharma JP, Rastogi V, Raghuvanshi RS, Moshiri M, Verma SP, Janus ED. Prevalence of coronary artery disease and coronary risk factors in rural and urban populations of north India. Eur Heart J 1997; 18:1728-1735.

46. Ramachandran A, Snehalatha C, Shyamala P, Vijay V, Viswanathan M. High prevalence of NIDDM and IGT in an elderly south Indian population with low rates of obesity. Diabetes Care 1994; 17:1190-1192.

47. Bhatnagar D, Anand IS, Durrington PN, Patel DJ, Wander GS, Mackness MI, Creed F, Tomenson B, Chandrashekhar Y, Winterbotham M. Coronary risk factors in people from the Indian subcontinent living in west London and their siblings in India. Lancet 1995; 345:405-409.

48. Ross R. Atherosclerosis--an inflammatory disease. N Engl J Med 1999; 340:115-126.

49. Chambers JC, Eda S, Bassett P, Karim Y, Thompson SG, Gallimore JR, Pepys MB, Kooner JS. C-reactive protein, insulin resistance, central obesity, and coronary heart disease risk in South Asians from the United Kingdom compared with White Europeans. Circulation 2001; 104:145-150.

50. Yudkin JS, Stehouwer CD, Emeis JJ, Coppack SW. C-reactive protein in healthy subjects: associations with obesity, insulin resistance, and endothelial dysfunction: a potential role for cytokines originating from adipose tissue? Arterioscler Thromb Vasc Biol 1999; 19:972-978.

51. Mohamed A, V, Goodrick S, Rawesh A, Katz DR, Miles JM, Yudkin JS, Klein S, Coppack SW. Subcutaneous adipose tissue releases interleukin-6, but not tumor necrosis factor-alpha, in vivo. J Clin Endocrinol Metab 1997; 82:4196-4200.

52. Chambers JC, Kooner JS. Homocysteine: a novel risk factor for coronary heart disease in UK South Asians. Heart 2001; 86:121-122.

53. Chambers JC, Ireland H, Thompson E, Reilly P, Obeid OA, Refsum H, Ueland P, Lane DA, Kooner JS. Methylenetetrahydrofolate reductase 677 C-->T mutation and coronary heart disease risk in UK South Asians. Arterioscler Thromb Vasc Biol 2000; 20:2448-2452.

54. Chambers JC, Ueland PM, Obeid OA, Wrigley J, Refsum H, Kooner JS. Improved vascular endothelial function after oral B vitamins: An effect mediated through reduced concentrations of free plasma homocysteine. Circulation 2000; 102:2479-2483.

55. Scanu AM. The role of lipoprotein(a) in the pathogenesis of atherosclerotic cardiovascular disease and its utility as predictor of coronary heart disease events. Curr Cardiol Rep 2001; 3:385-390.

56. Shlipak MG, Simon JA, Vittinghoff E, Lin F, Barrett-Connor E, Knopp RH, Levy RI, Hulley SB. Estrogen and progestin, lipoprotein(a), and the risk of recurrent coronary heart disease events after menopause. JAMA 2000; 283:1845-1852.

57. Evans RW, Shpilberg O, Shaten BJ, Ali S, Kamboh MI, Kuller LH. Prospective association of lipoprotein(a) concentrations and apo(a) size with coronary heart disease among men in the Multiple Risk Factor Intervention Trial. J Clin Epidemiol 2001; 54:51-57.

58. Boerwinkle E, Leffert CC, Lin J, Lackner C, Chiesa G, Hobbs HH. Apolipoprotein(a) gene accounts for greater than 90% of the variation in plasma lipoprotein(a) concentrations. J Clin Invest 1992; 90:52-60.

59.	Pati U, Pati N. Lipoprotein(a), atherosclerosis, and apolipoprotein(a) gene polymorphism. Mol Genet Metab 2000; 71:87-92.

60.	Low PS, Heng CK, Saha N, Tay JS. Racial variation of cord plasma lipoprotein(a) levels in relation to coronary risk level: a study in three ethnic groups in Singapore. Pediatr Res 1996; 40:718-722.

61.	Yajnik C. Interactions of perturbations in intrauterine growth and growth during childhood on the risk of adult-onset disease. Proc Nutr Soc 2000; 59:257-265.

62.	Steer P, Alam MA, Wadsworth J, Welch A. Relation between maternal haemoglobin concentration and birth weight in different ethnic groups. BMJ 1995; 310:489-491.

63.	Peabody JW, Gertler PJ, Leibowitz A. The policy implications of better structure and process on birth outcomes in Jamaica. Health Policy 1998; 43:1-13.

64.	Wen SW, Kramer MS, Usher RH. Comparison of birth weight distributions between Chinese and Caucasian infants. Am J Epidemiol 1995; 141:1177-1187.

65.	Caulfield LE, Harris SB, Whalen EA, Sugamori ME. Maternal nutritional status, diabetes and risk of macrosomia among Native Canadian women. Early Hum Dev 1998; 50:293-303.

66.	Stein CE, Fall CH, Kumaran K, Osmond C, Cox V, Barker DJ. Fetal growth and coronary heart disease in south India. Lancet 1996; 348:1269-1273.

67.	Barakat K, Stevenson S, Wilkinson P, Suliman A, Ranjadayalan K, Timmis AD. Socioeconomic differentials in recurrent ischaemia and mortality after acute myocardial infarction. Heart 2001; 85:390-394.

68.	Chaturvedi N, Rai H, Ben Shlomo Y. Lay diagnosis and health-care-seeking behaviour for chest pain in south Asians and Europeans . Lancet 1997; 350:1578-1583.

69.	Lear JT, Lawrence IG, Burden AC, Pohl JE. A comparison of stress test referral rates and outcome between Asians and Europeans. J R Soc Med 1994; 87:661-662.

70.	Lear JT, Lawrence IG, Pohl JE, Burden AC. Myocardial infarction and thrombolysis: a comparison of the Indian and European populations on a coronary care unit. J R Coll Physicians Lond 1994; 28:143-147.

71.	Dhawan J, Bray CL. Angiographic comparison of coronary artery disease between Asians and Caucasians. Postgrad Med J 1994; 70:625-630.

72.   Shaukat N, de Bono DP, Cruickshank JK. Clinical features, risk factors, and referral delay in British patients of Indian and European origin with angina matched for age and extent of coronary atheroma. BMJ 1993; 307:717-718.

73.   Kahn BB, Flier JS. Obesity and insulin resistance. J Clin Invest 2000; 106:473-481.

74.   Forouhi NG, Jenkinson G, Thomas EL, Mullick S, Mierisova S, Bhonsle U, McKeigue PM, Bell JD. Relation of triglyceride stores in skeletal muscle cells to central obesity and insulin sensitivity in European and South Asian men. Diabetologia 1999; 42:932-935.

75.   McKeigue PM, Pierpoint T, Ferrie JE, Marmot MG. Relationship of glucose intolerance and hyperinsulinaemia to body fat pattern in south Asians and Europeans. Diabetologia 1992; 35:785-791.

76.   Banerji MA, Faridi N, Atluri R, Chaiken RL, Lebovitz HE. Body composition, visceral fat, leptin, and insulin resistance in Asian Indian men. J Clin Endocrinol Metab 1999; 84:137-144.

77.   Trevisan M, Krogh V, Freudenheim J, Blake A, Muti P, Panico S, Farinaro E, Mancini M, Menotti A, Ricci G. Consumption of olive oil, butter, and vegetable oils and coronary heart disease risk factors. The Research Group ATS-RF2 of the Italian National Research Council. JAMA 1990; 263:688-692.

78.   Maron DJ, Fair JM, Haskell WL. Saturated fat intake and insulin resistance in men with coronary artery disease. The Stanford Coronary Risk Intervention Project Investigators and Staff. Circulation 1991; 84:2020-2027.

79.   Ascherio A, Rimm EB, Giovannucci EL, Spiegelman D, Stampfer M, Willett WC. Dietary fat and risk of coronary heart disease in men: cohort follow up study in the United States. BMJ 1996; 313:84-90.

80.   Snowdon DA, Phillips RL. Does a vegetarian diet reduce the occurrence of diabetes? Am J Public Health 1985; 75:507-512.

81.   Snowdon DA. Animal product consumption and mortality because of all causes combined, coronary heart disease, stroke, diabetes, and cancer in Seventh-day Adventists. Am J Clin Nutr 1988; 48 (Suppl):739-748.

82.   Kato H, Tillotson J, Nichaman MZ, Rhoads GG, Hamilton HB. Epidemiologic studies of coronary heart disease and stroke in Japanese men living in Japan, Hawaii and California. Am J Epidemiol 1973; 97:372-385.

83. Robertson TL, Kato H, Gordon T, Kagan A, Rhoads GG, Land CE, Worth RM, Belsky JL, Dock DS, Miyanishi M, Kawamoto S. Epidemiologic studies of coronary heart disease and stroke in Japanese men living in Japan, Hawaii and California. Coronary heart disease risk factors in Japan and Hawaii. Am J Cardiol 1977; 39:244-249.

84. McGee DL, Reed DM, Yano K, Kagan A, Tillotson J. Ten-year incidence of coronary heart disease in the Honolulu Heart Program. Relationship to nutrient intake. Am J Epidemiol 1984; 119:667-676.

85. Kushi LH, Lew RA, Stare FJ, Ellison CR, el Lozy M, Bourke G, Daly L, Graham I, Hickey N, Mulcahy R. Diet and 20-year mortality from coronary heart disease. The Ireland- Boston Diet-Heart Study. N Engl J Med 1985; 312:811-818.

86. Mann GV. Metabolic consequences of dietary trans fatty acids. Lancet 1994; 343:1268-1271.

87. Ascherio A, Willett WC. Metabolic and atherogenic effects of trans fatty acids. J Intern Med 1995; 238:93-96.

88. Christiansen E, Schnider S, Palmvig B, Tauber-Lassen E, Pedersen O. Intake of a diet high in trans monounsaturated fatty acids or saturated fatty acids. Effects on postprandial insulinemia and glycemia in obese patients with NIDDM. Diabetes Care 1997; 20:881-887.

89. Frost G, Leeds A, Trew G, Margara R, Dornhorst A. Insulin sensitivity in women at risk of coronary heart disease and the effect of a low glycemic diet. Metabolism 1998; 47:1245-1251.

90. Frost G, Keogh B, Smith D, Akinsanya K, Leeds A. The effect of low-glycemic carbohydrate on insulin and glucose response in vivo and in vitro in patients with coronary heart disease. Metabolism 1996; 45:669-672.

91. Lissin LW, Cooke JP. Phytoestrogens and cardiovascular health. J Am Coll Cardiol 2000; 35:1403-1410.

92. Anthony MS, Clarkson TB, Bullock BC, Wagner JD. Soy protein versus soy phytoestrogens in the prevention of diet-induced coronary artery atherosclerosis of male cynomolgus monkeys. Arterioscler Thromb Vasc Biol 1997; 17:2524-2531.

93. Sevak L, McKeigue PM, Marmot MG. Relationship of hyperinsulinemia to dietary intake in south Asian and European men. Am J Clin Nutr 1994; 59:1069-1074.

94. Singh RB, Ghosh S, Niaz AM, Gupta S, Bishnoi I, Sharma J, Agarwal P, Rastogi SS, Beegum R, Chibo H, Shoumin Z. Epidemiologic study of diet and

coronary risk factors in relation to central obesity and insulin levels in rural and urban populations of North India. Int J Cardiol 1995;47:245-255.

95. Helmrich SP, Ragland DR, Leung RW, Paffenbarger RS. Physical activity and reduced occurrence of non-insulin-dependent diabetes mellitus. N Engl J Med 1991; 325:147-152.

96. Wannamethee SG, Shaper AG, Alberti KG. Physical activity, metabolic factors, and the incidence of coronary heart disease and type 2 diabetes. Arch Intern Med 2000; 160:2108-2116.

97. Manson JE, Hu FB, Rich-Edwards JW, Colditz GA, Stampfer MJ, Willett WC, Speizer FE, Hennekens CH. A prospective study of walking as compared with vigorous exercise in the prevention of coronary heart disease in women. N Engl J Med 1999; 341:650-658.

98. Rodriguez BL, Curb JD, Burchfiel CM, Abbott RD, Petrovitch H, Masaki K, Chiu D. Physical activity and 23-year incidence of coronary heart disease morbidity and mortality among middle-aged men. The Honolulu Heart Program. Circulation 1994; 89:2540-2544.

99. Fletcher GF, Balady G, Blair SN, Blumenthal J, Caspersen C, Chaitman B, Epstein S, Sivarajan Froelicher ES, Froelicher VF, Pina IL, Pollock ML. Statement on exercise: benefits and recommendations for physical activity programs for all Americans. A statement for health professionals by the Committee on Exercise and Cardiac Rehabilitation of the Council on Clinical Cardiology, American Heart Association. Circulation 1996; 94:857-862.

100. Tuomilehto J, Lindstrom J, Eriksson JG, Valle TT, Hamalainen H, Ilanne-Parikka P, Keinanen-Kiukaanniemi S, Laakso M, Louheranta A, Rastas M, Salminen V, Uusitupa M. Prevention of type 2 diabetes mellitus by changes in lifestyle among subjects with impaired glucose tolerance. N Engl J Med 2001; 344:1343-1350.

101. Stern MP. Strategies and prospects for finding insulin resistance genes. J Clin Invest 2000; 106:323-327.

102. Duggirala R, Blangero J, Almasy L, Arya R, Dyer TD, Williams KL, Leach RJ, O'Connell P, Stern MP . A major locus for fasting insulin concentrations and insulin resistance on chromosome 6q with strong pleiotropic effects on obesity-related phenotypes in nondiabetic Mexican Americans. Am J Hum Genet 2001; 68:1149-1164.

103. Maddux BA, Sbraccia P, Kumakura S, Sasson S, Youngren J, Fisher A, Spencer S, Grupe A, Henzel W, Stewart TA, et a. Membrane glycoprotein PC-1 and insulin resistance in non-insulin-dependent diabetes mellitus. Nature 1995; 373:448-451.

104. Goldfine ID, Maddux BA, Youngren JF, Frittitta L, Trischitta V, Dohm GL. Membrane glycoprotein PC-1 and insulin resistance. Mol Cell Biochem 1998; 182:177-184.

105. Schumacher MC, Hasstedt SJ, Hunt SC, Williams RR, Elbein SC. Major gene effect for insulin levels in familial NIDDM pedigrees. Diabetes 1992; 41:416-423.

106. Kooner JS, Baliga RR, Wilding J, Crook D, Packard CJ, Banks LM, Peart S, Aitman TJ, Scott J. Abdominal obesity, impaired nonesterified fatty acid suppression, and insulin-mediated glucose disposal are early metabolic abnormalities in families with premature myocardial infarction. Arterioscler Thromb Vasc Biol 1998; 18:1021-1026.

107. Cassell PG, Saker PJ, Huxtable SJ, Kousta E, Jackson AE, Hattersley AT, Frayling TM, Walker M, Kopelman PG, Ramachandran A, Snehelatha C, Hitman GA, McCarthy MI. Evidence that single nucleotide polymorphism in the uncoupling protein 3 (UCP3) gene influences fat distribution in women of European and Asian origin. Diabetologia 2000; 43:1558-1564.

108. Effect of intensive blood-glucose control with metformin on complications in overweight patients with type 2 diabetes (UKPDS 34). UK Prospective Diabetes Study (UKPDS) Group. Lancet 1998; 352:854-865.

109. Intensive blood-glucose control with sulphonylureas or insulin compared with conventional treatment and risk of complications in patients with type 2 diabetes (UKPDS 33). UK Prospective Diabetes Study (UKPDS) Group. Lancet 1998; 352:837-853.

110. Weinstock RS, Dai H, Wadden TA. Diet and exercise in the treatment of obesity: effects of 3 interventions on insulin resistance . Arch Intern Med 1998; 158:2477-2483.

111. Ross R, Dagnone D, Jones PJ, Smith H, Paddags A, Hudson R, Janssen I. Reduction in obesity and related comorbid conditions after diet-induced weight loss or exercise-induced weight loss in men. A randomized, controlled trial. Ann Intern Med 2000; 133:92-103.

112. Antonucci T, Whitcomb R, McLain R, Lockwood D, Norris RM. Impaired glucose tolerance is normalized by treatment with the thiazolidinedione troglitazone. Diabetes Care 1997; 20:188-193.

113. Schoonjans K, Auwerx J. Thiazolidinediones: an update. Lancet 2000; 355:1008-1010.

114. Kendall A, Levitsky DA, Strupp BJ, Lissner L. Weight loss on a low-fat diet: consequence of the imprecision of the control of food intake in humans. Am J Clin Nutr 1991; 53:1124-1129.

115. McKeigue PM, Marmot MG, Adelstein AM, Hunt SP, Shipley MJ, Butler SM, Riemersma RA, Turner PR. Diet and risk factors for coronary heart disease in Asians in northwest London. Lancet 1985; 2:1086-1090.

116. Beegom R, Beegom R, Niaz MA, Singh RB. Diet, central obesity and prevalence of hypertension in the urban population of south India. Int J Cardiol 1995; 51:183-191.

117. Pais P, Pogue J, Gerstein H, Zachariah E, Savitha D, Jayprakash S, Nayak PR, Yusuf S. Risk factors for acute myocardial infarction in Indians: a case- control study. Lancet 1996; 348:358-363.

118. National Service Framework for Coronary Heart Disease. HMSO, London. 2000.

119. Harper CR, Jacobson TA. New perspectives on the management of low levels of high-density lipoprotein cholesterol. Arch Intern Med 1999; 159:1049-1057.

120. Rubins HB, Robins SJ, Collins D, Fye CL, Anderson JW, Elam MB, Faas FH, Linares E, Schaefer EJ, Schectman G, Wilt TJ, Wittes J. Gemfibrozil for the secondary prevention of coronary heart disease in men with low levels of high-density lipoprotein cholesterol. Veterans Affairs High-Density Lipoprotein Cholesterol Intervention Trial Study Group. N Engl J Med 1999; 341:410-418.

121. Assmann G, Schulte H, von Eckardstein A. Hypertriglyceridemia and elevated lipoprotein(a) are risk factors for major coronary events in middle-aged men. Am J Cardiol 1996; 77:1179-1184.

122. van den Hoogen PC, Feskens EJ, Nagelkerke NJ, Menotti A, Nissinen A, Kromhout D. The relation between blood pressure and mortality due to coronary heart disease among men in different parts of the world. Seven Countries Study Research Group. N Engl J Med 2000; 342:1-8.

123. Kaplan NM. Systolic hypertension in the elderly program (SHEP) and Swedish trial in old patients with hypertension (STOP). The promises and the potential problems. Am J Hypertens 1992; 5:331-334.

124. Hansson L, Zanchetti A, Carruthers SG, Dahlof B , Elmfeldt D, Julius S, Menard J, Rahn KH, Wedel H , Westerling S. Effects of intensive blood-pressure lowering and low-dose aspirin in patients with hypertension: principal results of the Hypertension Optimal Treatment (HOT) randomised trial. HOT Study Group. Lancet 1998; 351:1755-1762.

125. Anderson KM, Odell PM, Wilson PW, Kannel WB. Cardiovascular disease risk profiles. Am Heart J 1991; 121(1 Pt 2):293-298.

126. Grundy SM, Pasternak R, Greenland P, Smith S, Jr., Fuster V. Assessment of cardiovascular risk by use of multiple-risk-factor assessment equations: a statement for healthcare professionals from the American Heart Association and the American College of Cardiology. Circulation 1999; 100:1481-1492.

127. Wood D, De Backer G, Faergeman O, Graham I, Mancia G, Pyorala K. Prevention of coronary heart disease in clinical practice: recommendations of the Second Joint Task Force of European and other Societies on Coronary Prevention. Atherosclerosis 1998; 140:199-270.

128. Joint British recommendations on prevention of coronary heart disease in clinical practice: summary. British Cardiac Society, British Hyperlipidaemia Association, British Hypertension Society, British Diabetic Association. BMJ 2000; 320:705-708.

129. Leaverton PE, Sorlie PD, Kleinman JC, Dannenberg AL, Ingster-Moore L, Kannel WB, Cornoni-Huntley JC. Representativeness of the Framingham risk model for coronary heart disease mortality: a comparison with a national cohort study. J Chronic Dis 1987; 40:775-784.

130. Brand RJ, Rosenman RH, Sholtz RI, Friedman M. Multivariate prediction of coronary heart disease in the Western Collaborative Group Study compared to the findings of the Framingham study . Circulation 1976; 53:348-355.

131. Relationship of blood pressure, serum cholesterol, smoking habit, relative weight and ECG abnormalities to incidence of major coronary events: final report of the pooling project. The pooling project research group. J Chronic Dis 1978; 31:201-306.

132. Baseline risk factors and their association with outcome in the West of Scotland Coronary Prevention Study. The West of Scotland Coronary Prevention Study Group [see comments]. Am J Cardiol 1997; 79:756-762.

133. Chambless LE, Dobson AJ, Patterson CC, Raines B . On the use of a logistic risk score in predicting risk of coronary heart disease. Stat Med 1990; 9:385-396.

134. Chambers JC, Wrigley J, Kooner JS. Evaluation of the Joint British Societies coronary heart disease risk calculator in UK South Asians. Heart 2000; 83 (suppl):43A.

3

Coronary heart disease in South Asians: the impact of diabetes mellitus

J K Cruickshank, A Vyas, M Banerjee and J C Oldroyd

Introduction

The key question posed by the title of this chapter is: "How much of the excess coronary heart disease (CHD) in populations of South Asian origin is related or even 'due' to glucose intolerance or overt type 2 diabetes, with all the heterogeneity of culture, current geography and different environments"? Unfortunately, adequate data are not yet available to answer the question even approximately, mainly because cohorts of adequate sample size are not yet available. However, the difficulty is also in part because the notion of what diabetes is as a diagnostic entity is beginning to change and also because of the slow realisation that its metabolic precursors develop early in life (see chapter 4). Excess diabetes continues to be a public health issue across all South Asian sub-groups in Britain since it was first described in 1980 and in the several surveys since [1-8]. Looking at the British reports, a key point that recurs throughout the literature is that the excess of diabetes, and frequently its prodrome, glucose intolerance, is also accompanied by a variety of other risk factor differences compared with those individuals still apparently normoglycaemic, South Asian or not, who remain at risk of developing these conditions later.

Another way of posing this chapter's question more technically is to ask, what is the population attributable risk from the upward shift in the blood glucose distribution of South Asians for incident coronary heart disease? The ideal would be to compare outcomes of South Asian people with and without diabetes with the experience of other populations. Again, unfortunately, such data are scarce in any population. The best dataset for such comparison remains the largest available, with outcomes now 20 years since the original classification of men from the MRFIT study[9]. Where results for "South Asians" would lie on this plot is unknown.

Figure 3.1 Age adjusted Cardiovascular death rates by systolic blood pressure (or other risk factors) for men with and without diabetes at initial screening for MRFIT (adapted from ref 9).

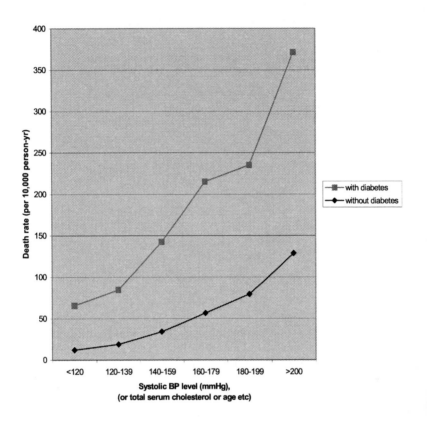

The global nature of diabetes among South Asians

Diabetes is a global problem among people of South Asian origin, as previously noted in the mid 20th Century in the Caribbean[10], South Africa[11], Fiji[12], and more recently in Mauritius[13]. Data from the subcontinent itself has begun to show similar high rates of diabetes[14]. Worryingly and perhaps surprisingly, in our comparison of British migrants from specific villages in Gujarat and people still resident in the same semi-rural area of origin there, rates of glucose intolerance and known diabetes were as high in India as in the UK population samples at some 15%. However, unlike other key underlying CHD risk factors, glucose intolerance was the only one not to be greatly increased in the migrants, in whom for example body mass indices were a mean of 5 kg/m^2 greater (*paper submitted*). Possibly, lifestyle changes had already been in process for these 'villagers' so that their body mass indices, despite apparently still being 'low' at means of 21.5 kg/m^2, were higher than appropriate for their body build and current local setting, perhaps in part because physical activity undertaken was less than that experienced 10 years earlier. Life and facilities had certainly changed over the previous decade in the greatly expanded and now bustling, traffic-hindered township around which their villages were located. These data suggest that most of the excess vascular risk conferred on Indian migrants compared with their contemporaries still in their Indian villages of origin is due to substantial increases in standard risk factors, that is adiposity, high blood pressure and dyslipidaemia.

CHD in Diabetes itself

In people already diagnosed with diabetes, very few studies have been conducted specifically to examine excess CHD risk, if any, associated with 'South Asian' ethnicity. An early report from Leicester, UK did find that the relatively high and excess CHD rate in mainly Gujarati people there was associated with diabetes but was not accounted for entirely by such known diabetes[15]. However, as the data were collected after the CHD event, the role of prior glucose intolerance and unknown diabetes could not be estimated. The UK Prospective Diabetes Study found slightly but not significantly higher age standardized rates for fatal and non- fatal myocardial infarction amongst South Asians with type 2 diabetes (15.4 (95%CI 10.6 –21.4) per 1000 person years) compared with whites, 14.6 (13.3 to 15.9), and African-Caribbeans, 4.3 (2.5-7.0)[16], although this was attenuated after adjustment for conventional risk factors.

Causes of the excess glucose intolerance

The causes of the excess glucose intolerance remain unclear. Insulin insensitivity or resistance, a descriptive term which throws little or no light on the aetiology of the hyperglycaemia (see section below), is a widespread finding and, together with actual levels of blood glucose, predicts those more likely to develop later diabetes, in South Asian and other populations. However, contrary to an initial hypothesis, insulin resistance does not predict later CHD consistently in any population, and most particularly not at all to date in the three disparate Indian origin populations studied, 2 in London ([17] and Gandi & McKeigue 8 year follow up, 1999 unpublished, but presented at 'Heart Health in Developing Countries' conference, Delhi October 1999) and the other large sample in Mauritius (Tuomilehto et al

2000 – unpublished manuscript, personal communication. (*Note publication bias here: 2 of 3 negative studies still unpublished*).

Body fat, general and early life factors

However, as in any other population, critical factors underlying diabetes development in South Asians include: body fat accumulation whether as rising BMI (at levels as low as or lower than 22 kg/m^2), or as a particular propensity to increased abdominal fat, measured as waist alone or as waist/hip or waist/thigh circumference ratios; energy imbalance as inadequate energy expenditure from too little general physical activity for given dietary intakes. Increased abdominal fat falls under the umbrella of another vague but highly fashionable term, the 'metabolic syndrome'. This includes insulin resistance and concurrent glucose intolerance, dyslipidaemia, 'hypertension' (variably defined) and increasingly other concomitant, more recent metabolic risk factors. How much morbidity or mortality the syndrome *per se* contributes over and above its component risk factors is unclear. Nevertheless, the syndrome is of course commoner in South Asians compared with western populations[18,19]. Risk factors for developing the metabolic syndrome, in South Asians particularly, may include the use of ghee and the consumption of low amounts of all of the following: vitamin C, vitamin E, omega –3 fatty acids especially eicosapentanoic (EPA) and docosapentanoic (DHA), and monounsaturated fatty acids[19]. Lower birth weight has been associated with a high prevalence of the metabolic syndrome in later life[20] and small birth dimensions are also found in South Asians compared with other ethnic groups, a finding that seems to persist in subsequent generations to date to date[21], as we have found across ethnic subgroups from the subcontinent in a national dataset[22]. Low initial body size, in addition to excess catch-up growth and greater BMI during childhood, may increase risk of any glucose intolerance and later overt 'diabetes'. This is perhaps amongst the best-studied example of the Hales/Barker 'thrifty phenotype' hypothesis (as discussed later by Fall in chapter 5).

Recently Yajnik has shown that in babies of mothers in Pune, India, insulin concentrations in cord blood were raised compared with that of white European babies born in London and were correlated with sub-scapular skinfold thicknesses[23]. His follow-up studies have also shown that later in childhood these 'thin-fat' Indian babies become more insulin resistant[24], an association that is modified by postnatal growth: greater catch up growth results in greater insulin resistance. This needs further investigation if only to clarify definitions of catch up growth (length, weight, head circumference, central fat).

Other nutritional factors

The role of raised blood homocysteine (Hcy) levels among South Asians, with or without diabetes, is currently being investigated widely. At a molecular level, Hcy facilitates oxidant injury to the vascular endothelium and inhibits nitric oxide production, thus promoting atherosclerosis and coronary heart disease. A meta-analysis found that Hcy concentrations that were 25% lower than average were associated with a lower risk of CHD (OR 0.89, 95% CI 0.89 to 0.96) and stroke (OR 0.81, 95% 0.68 to 0.95) compared with normal Hcy concentrations[25]. Recent studies have shown that plasma Hcy concentrations are higher in adult British South Asians than white Europeans[26, 27]. Dietary supplements of folate and vitamin B_{12} have been shown to reduce plasma Hcy concentrations by up to 25%. Nutritional factors are likely to be important since reduced intake of vitamin B_{12} and folate, due to prolonged cooking of vegetables (which may destroy up to 90% of folate), have been reported in Gujaratis[28]. Our own data have found very low dietary folate intakes in Indians living in Indian villages. Perhaps surprisingly, raised Hcy is found both in the sub-continent itself, and in migrant people and their descendents abroad. The simultaneous presence of excesses of some and deficiency of other specific dietary fatty acids, e.g. long chain polyunsaturates such as EPA and DHA acid (as found in oily fish), is another continuing area of research.

Endothelial dysfunction, arising from oxidative damage due to glucose intolerance and from diets low in antioxidants or hyperhomocysteinaemia, results in an increased expression of inflammatory molecules such as cytokines (e.g. interleukin 6, which is also released from adipose tissue). Cytokines, which predict myocardial infarction in healthy men[29], stimulate the liver to release the acute phase reactant C reactive protein (CRP), an inflammatory marker. CRP concentration is itself a sensitive predictor of first CVD events[28]. Based on pilot studies in Manchester, CRP levels are higher in Pakistanis[31] and in British Gujaratis than in comparable European populations, with lower levels in UK African-Caribbeans[31], whose CHD risk is lowest. Elevated CRP has also been associated with higher serum insulin and glycosylated haemoglobin (HbA1c) concentrations, suggesting a possible role of inflammation in insulin resistance and glucose intolerance[32].

Genetic and environmental interactions in insulin resistance

Many nutritional factors and body composition changes over the life span, and how these factors may transmit risk across generations, remain to be explored, potentially with considerable importance for public health for South Asian communities. As yet, despite considerable searching, no geno-phenotypic clues or 'candidate genes' have been discovered to underlie the South Asian diabetes excess. In the authors' view, this remains less likely than transmitted intergenerational risk (see below).

1. *Energy balance*: In this context energy balance is critical, that is the balance between dietary energy consumed and metabolic energy expended, both basal and then that required to power physical activity. If net balance becomes positive, weight gain results (and generally persists, unless extra activity expends it!). Very few studies have measured physical activity among South Asian or other ethnic groups, not least because reliable methods for doing so in free-living individuals have only recently begun to become available. The untested hypothesis is that for specific body sizes or weight, South Asian groups tend to have less muscle mass and hence less surface area on which insulin can act to dispose of (excess) dietary energy, even for given levels of physical activity. Apparent and real insulin 'resistance' will occur. If physical activity is also lower at given levels of energy intake, then positive energy balance must follow, leading to weight gain. To the current authors, such a hypothesis relating energy *balance* over the life-course with as yet generally lower muscle fibre number and bulk from smaller initial body size is much more likely a causal background to later glucose intolerance and CHD than inherent 'insulin resistance', which we would suggest is entirely secondary to these predisposing factors and not otherwise inherent.

2. *An intergenerational, non-genetic hypothesis:* The intriguing sequel that logically follows is that inherent diabetes and CHD risk in these communities must then be genetic. We would point out that while a few polymorphic genetic markers have been identified that may be more common in South Asian populations, including related to factor VII clotting activity[33] and to the MTFHR gene variants ([34]ATVB 1999), very few have as yet been

repeatedly linked to either the 'diabetes' or CHD phenotype in any population. We would suggest the apparently inherent risk of both 'diabetes' and CHD is more likely to be transmitted by intergenerational mechanisms due to repeated environmental exposures rather than inherent genomic variants. For example during pregnancy in women of relatively small stature, mild 'hyperglycaemia' and minor variations in concurrent metabolic factors such as specific and total fatty acid concentrations may be present as yet unrecognized as outside the usual range for that habitus. It is well-established that in gestational or pre-pregnancy type 2 diabetes, levels of insulin in amniotic fluid are elevated, associated with increased cord blood insulin levels in the infant[35]. Such small persistent metabolic variations may well therefore transmit through generations due to external not genetic causes. Direct tests of these issues are underway in our maternal-infant studies.

3. *Ethnic sub-group similarity or heterogeneity*: South Asians of most ethnic sub-groups appear to be susceptible to the diabetes and CHD syndromes. Sub-groups include Hindu or Muslim, vegetarian or omnivore, Gujarati, Sikh, Bangladeshi or Pakistani or any other method of describing the religious, dietary, geographic and hence cultural diversity across the subcontinent and its migrants and their descendants abroad. However, if small initial size at birth (a universal feature to date compared with other western populations), relatively low muscle fibre number which increases little after birth, as well as lower overall muscle mass and variable catch-up growth, followed for those of adequate financial means by generally excess dietary energy intake in later life, the underlying phenotype will be similar across the ethnic sub-groups. Yajnik's[23, 24] and Fall's work, outlined elsewhere in this volume, illustrate the potential for these issues to apply.

A critique of 'Insulin Resistance'

Finally, it is worth examining the validity and credibility of the insulin resistance hypothesis for CHD, because it has been applied with such vigour to the CHD problem among South Asians. Simplistically, insulin resistance can be defined as excess plasma insulin for given plasma glucose levels – which would be lower if insulin action were as effective as 'usual'. Insulin resistance is apparently commoner in South Asians and as such has been floated as the major mechanism underlying the reported excess of both diabetes and CHD[36]. This suggestion has many flaws, which are outlined below and build on a previous comment[37], including 2 immediate caveats to any such definitions of insulin resistance. These are:

1. *Peripheral venous blood measures*: Note that to define insulin resistance, what is universally measured are peripheral _venous_ plasma levels of both 'insulin' and glucose, and *not arterial* levels. Arterial blood levels are the circulating concentrations that all tissues respond to apart from the liver, right heart, lung alveoli and their vascular endothelia, as insulin is secreted into pancreatic venous, flowing into portal, blood. Measuring arterial or portal venous blood is not widely possible, hence nor is what really influences peripheral blood insulin levels – insulin's 'first pass' hepatic uptake, known to be highly variable depending on fasting or fed status, time since last meal and that meal's composition etc.

2. *Assay specificity*: a second critical technical point is how insulin is assayed. Most studies have measured 'insulin' using a traditional radioimmunoassay with a widely available polyclonal antibody, which has major if variable cross-reactivity with its pro-insulin precursor molecule. When specific monoclonal antibodies against 'intact insulin', pro-insulin and its split product, 32-33 split pro-insulin are used in respective assays, 10-20% of apparent insulin in the traditional assay is found to be these other molecules[38].

3. *Pro- and Split Pro- Insulins:* Apart from the possibility that pro-insulin itself and 32-33 split pro-insulin may have direct toxic actions on vascular endothelium and beta-cells, the variable proportions of pro-insulins also likely compete with intact insulin at its receptor, leading to apparent 'resistance'. Intriguingly, in 2 recent cohort analyses, when pro-insulin or 32-33 were measured as well as insulin, they displaced insulin itself in predicting diabetes[39, 40]. In a third, among adolescents followed from birth, pro-insulin levels were more closely correlated with early life indices than was insulin[41].

4. *Problems with interpreting clamp studies*: A further major problem of interpretation in studies of insulin resistance is physiological and comes in 'clamp' studies, regarded by biochemical investigators as the gold standard test. By definition, physiological insulin release and its control are primarily driven by food intake, hence gastric filling

itself and the nature of the food consumed (simple or more complex sugars primarily, fatty and amino acids etc.). Clamp studies entirely bypass this entero-hepatic circulation and their physiological relevance remains uncertain, if not always to those doing them.

5. *The IGF system and its binding proteins:* Key influences on sensitivity in liver cells to (intact) insulin in portal blood are type and quantity of fatty acids, which are continuously released from visceral fat but also rise substantially after meals, and render hepatic cellular responses much less sensitive to insulin (= hepatic insulin resistance). Hence recent, 'acute' dietary composition and what is derived 'chronically' from the diet over the longer term but stored as visceral fat are key effectors. In this context, other insulin-like molecules are important, notably the insulin-like growth factors (IGF) and their several binding proteins (IGF-BP), themselves biologically and possibly vasoactive. IGF-I has insulin-like actions cross-reacting with the insulin receptor, while IGFBP-1, its main tissue-release modifier, is synthesized in non-pregnant human beings only by the liver where its release is tightly but negatively regulated by portal blood insulin. IGFBP-1 hence also seems to be closely regulated by portal blood fatty acid concentrations. Finally, there are major variations in serum IGF system concentrations by ethnic group as we have described[42], and these not only relate to cardiovascular risk in cross-sectional study[43] but also longitudinally predict development of overt diabetes[44].

Conclusion

This discussion illustrates the many current themes under investigation, often somewhat confusingly at varying points along potential causal pathways leading to the disease endpoints. No direct evidence as yet supports efforts specifically aimed just at prevention for South Asian populations. However, general measures, which are beginning to be found to work generally, apply even more so to any South Asian community, in general public health terms.

Public Health action: Control of hyperglycaemia or overt diabetes is a separate topic but aggressive management of hyperglycaemia before diabetes is diagnosed by life style measures is effective in delaying and possibly preventing overt diabetes[45,46]. Importantly, lifestyle interventions for the prevention of diabetes have not been tested in South Asians in the UK. After formal diagnosis of diabetes, aggressive management of standard risk factors seems clearly indicated although some authors have suggested that pre-diabetes care is appropriate in South Asians[47]. This applies particularly to (high) blood pressure and lipidaemia, probably below levels accepted for other ethnic groups because of the increased cardiovascular risk[48].

These types of measures should help to contain the global public health problem of diabetes and its vascular sequelae in South Asian populations, even without adequate explanations of the excess of either condition as yet. Major research efforts are and need to be underway to resolve the issues, which should throw light on the aetiology of these epidemics for everyone.

References

1. Cruickshank JK, Beevers DG, Osbourne VL, Haynes RA, Corlett JC, Selby S. Heart attack, stroke, diabetes and hypertension in West Indians, Asians and whites in Birmingham, England. BMJ 1997; 281:1108.

2. Mather HM, Keen H. The Southall Diabetes Survey: prevalence of known diabetes in Asians and Europeans. British Medical Journal 1985; 291:1081-1084.

3. McKeigue PM, Marmot MG, Syndercombe-Court YD, Cottier DE, Rahman S, Riemersma RA. Diabetes, hyperinsulinaemia, and coronary risk factors in Bangladeshis in East London. Br Heart J 1988; 60:390-396.

4. Simmons D., Williams DR, Powell MJ. Prevalence of diabetes in a predominantly Asian community: preliminary findings of the Coventry diabetes study. BMJ 1989; 298:18-21.

5. McKeigue PM, Shah B, Marmot MG. Relation of central obesity and insulin resistance with high diabetes prevalence and cardiovascular risk in South Asians. Lancet 1991; 337:382-386.

6. Cruickshank JK, Cooper J, Burnett M, Macduff J, Drubra U. Ethnic differences in fasting plasma C-peptide and insulin in relation to glucose tolerance and blood pressure. Lancet 1991; 338:842-847.

7. Bhopal R, Unwin N, White M, Yallop J, Walker L, Alberti KG et al. Heterogeneity of coronary heart disease risk factors in Indian, Pakistani, Bangladeshi and European origin populations: cross sectional study. BMJ 1999; 319:215-220.

8.   Riste L, Khan F, Cruickshank K. High prevalence of type 2 diabetes in all ethnic groups, including Europeans, in a British inner city: relative poverty, history, inactivity, or 21st century Europe? Diabetes Care 2001; 24:1377-1383.

9.   Stamler J, Vaccaro O, Neaton JD, Wentworth D. Diabetes, other risk factors, and 12-yr cardiovascular mortality for men screened in the Multiple Risk Factor Intervention Trial. Diabetes Care. 1993;16:434-44.

10.   Poon-King T, Henry M, Rampersad F. Prevalence and natural history of diabetes in Trinidad. Lancet 1968;1:155-9.

11.   Omar MA, Seedat MA, Dyer RB, Motala AA, Knight LT, Becker PJ. South African Indians show a high prevalence of NIDDM and bimodality in plasma glucose distribution patterns. Diabetes Care 1994;17:70-3.

12.   Zimmet P, Taylor R, Ram P, King H, Sloman G, Raper LR et al. Prevalence of diabetes and impaired glucose tolerance in the biracial (Melanesian and Indian) population of Fiji: a rural-urban comparison. Am.J.Epidemiol. 1983;118:673-88.

13.   Dowse GK, Zimmet PZ, King H. Relationship between prevalence of impaired glucose tolerance and NIDDM in a population. Diabetes Care 1991;14:968-74.

14.   Deepa R, Shanthi RS, Premalatha G, Mohan V. Comparison of ADA 1997 and WHO 1985 criteria for diabetes in south Indians--the Chennai Urban Population Study. American Diabetes Association. Diabet.Med. 2000;17:872-4.

15.   Woods KL, Samanta A, Burden AC. Diabetes mellitus as a risk factor for acute myocardial infarction in Asians and Europeans. Br Heart J. 1989;62:118-22.

16.   UKPDS. Ethnicity and cardiovascular disease. The incidence of myocardial infarction in white, South Asian, and Afro-Caribbean patients with type 2 diabetes (U.K. Prospective Diabetes Study 32). Diabetes Care 1998;21:1271-7.

17.   Yudkin JS, Denver AE, Mohamed-Ali V, Ramaiya KL, Nagi DK, Goubet S et al. The relationship of concentrations of insulin and proinsulin-like molecules with coronary heart disease prevalence and incidence; a study of two ethnic groups. Diabetes-Care 1997; 20:1093-1100.

18.   Das UN. Metabolic syndrome X is common in South Asians, but why and how? Nutrition 2002; 18: 774-6.

19.   Das UN. Nutritional deficiencies and the prevalence of syndrome X in South Asians. Nutrition 2002;18:282.

20.   Barker DJ, Hales CN, Fall CH, Osmond C, Phipps K, Clark PM. Type 2 (non-insulin-dependent) diabetes mellitus, hypertension and hyperlipidaemia (syndrome X): relation to reduced fetal growth. Diabetologia 1993;36:62-7.

21.   Margetts BM, Mohd YS, Al Dallal Z, Jackson AA. Persistence of lower birth weight in second generation South Asian babies born in the United Kingdom. J.Epidemiol.Community Health 2002;56:684-7.

22.   Harding S, Rosato MG, Cruickshank JK. Lack of change in birth weights of infants by generational status among Indian, Pakistani, Bangladeshi, Black Caribbean and Black African mothers in a British cohort study. Int J Epidemiol 2004 (in press).

23.   Yajnik CS, Lubree HG, Rege SS, Naik SS, Deshpande JA, Deshpande SS et al. Adiposity and hyperinsulinemia in Indians are present at birth. J.Clin.Endocrinol.Metab 2002;87:5575-80.

24.   Yajnik CS, Fall CH, Coyaji KJ, Hirve SS, Rao S, Barker DJ, Joglekar C, Kellingray S. Neonatal anthropometry: the thin-fat Indian baby. The Pune Maternal Nutrition Study. Int J Obes Relat Metab Disord. 2003;27:173-80.

25.   The Homocysteine Studies Collaboration. Homocysteine and risk of ischemic heart disease and stroke: a meta-analysis. JAMA 2002;288:2015-22.

26.   Chambers JC, Obeid OA, Refsum H, Ueland P, Hackett D, Hooper J et al. Plasma homocysteine concentrations and risk of coronary heart disease in UK Indian Asian and European men. Lancet 2000;355:523-7.

27.   Obeid OA, Mannan N, Perry G, Iles RA, Boucher BJ. Homocysteine and folate in healthy east London Bangladeshis. Lancet 1998;352:1829-30.

28.   Abraham R, Brown MC, North WR, McFadyen IR. Diets of Asian pregnant women in Harrow: iron and vitamins. Hum.Nutr.Appl.Nutr. 1987;41:164-73.

29.   Ridker PM, Rifai N, Stampfer MJ, Hennekens CH. Plasma concentration of interleukin-6 and the risk of future myocardial infarction among apparently healthy men. Circulation 2000; 101:1767-72.

30.   Ridker PM, Rifai N, Rose L, Buring JE, Cook NR. Comparison of C-reactive protein and low-density lipoprotein cholesterol levels in the prediction of first cardiovascular events. NEJM. 2002;347:1557-65.

31.   Heald AH, Anderson SG, Ivison F, Laing I, Gibson JM, Cruickshank K. C-reactive protein and the insulin-like growth factor (IGF)-system in relation to risk of cardiovascular disease in different ethnic groups. Atherosclerosis. 2003;170:79-86.

32. Wu T, Dorn JP, Donahue RP, Sempos CT, Trevisan M. Associations of serum C-reactive protein with fasting insulin, glucose, and glycosylated hemoglobin: the Third National Health and Nutrition Examination Survey, 1988-1994. American Journal of Epidemiology. 2002;155:65-71.

33. Lane A, Cruickshank JK, Stewart A, Henderson A, Humphries S, Green F. Genetic and Environmental Determinants of Factor VII Coagulant Activity in Ethnic Groups at Differing Risk of Coronary Heart Disease. Atherosclerosis 1992; 94: 43-50.

34. Chambers JC, Ireland H, Thompson E, Reilly P, Obeid OA, Refsum H, Ueland P, Lane DA, Kooner JS. Methylenetetrahydrofolate reductase 677 C-->T mutation and coronary heart disease risk in UK Indian Asians. Arterioscler Thromb Vasc Biol. 2000;20:2448-52.

35. Silverman BL, Rizzo T, Green OC, Cho NH, Winter RJ, Ogata ES, Richards GE, Metzger BE. Long-term prospective evaluation of offspring of diabetic mothers. Diabetes. 1991;40 Suppl 2:121-5.

36. McKeigue PM, Ferrie JE, Pierpoint T, Marmot MG. Association of early-onset coronary heart disease in South Asian men with glucose intolerance and hyperinsulinemia. Circulation. 1993;87:152-61.

37. JKCruickshank Challenging the orthodoxy of insulin resistance. Lancet. 1995;346:772-3.

38. Davies MJ, Metcalfe J, Day JL, Grenfell A, Hales CN, Gray IP. Effect of sulphonylurea therapy on plasma insulin, intact and 32/33 split proinsulin in subjects with type 2 diabetes mellitus. Diabet Med. 1994;11:293-8.

39. Wareham NJ, Byrne CD, Williams R, Day NE, Hales CN. Fasting proinsulin concentrations predict the development of type 2 diabetes. Diabetes Care. 1999;22:262-70.

40. Zethelius B, Byberg L, Hales CN, Lithell H, Berne C. Proinsulin is an independent predictor of coronary heart disease: Report from a 27-year follow-up study. Circulation. 2002;105:2153-8.

41. Singhal A, Fewtrell M, Cole TJ, Lucas A. Low nutrient intake and early growth for later insulin resistance in adolescents born preterm. Lancet. 2003;361:1089-97.

42. Cruickshank JK, Heald AH, Anderson SG, Cade JE, SampayoJ, Riste LK, Greenhalgh A, Taylor W, Fraser W, White A & Gibson JM. The epidemiology of the Insulin-like Growth Factor system in three ethnic groups. Am J Epidem 2001: 154: 504-513.

43. Heald AH, Cruickshank JK, Riste LK, Cade JE, Anderson S, Greenhalgh A, Sampayo J, Taylor W, Fraser W, White A, Gibson JM. Close relation of fasting insulin-like growth

factor binding protein-1 (IGFBP-1) with glucose tolerance and cardiovascular risk in two populations. Diabetologia 2001; 44: 333-9.

44.   Sandhu M, Heald A, Gibson M, Cruickshank JK, Dunger D, Wareham N. Circulating concentrations of insulin like growth factor-1 and development of glucose intolerance: a prospective observational study. Lancet 2002; 359: 1740-45.

45.   Tuomilehto J, Lindstrom J, Eriksson J,G, Valle TT, Hamalainen H, Ilanne-Parikka P et al . Prevention of type 2 diabetes mellitus by changes in lifestyle among subjects with impaired glucose tolerance. N.Engl.J.Med. 2001; 344: 1343-50.

46.   Knowler WC, Barrett-Connor E, Fowler SE, Hamman RF, Lachin JM, Walker EA et al. Reduction in the incidence of type 2 diabetes with lifestyle intervention or metformin. N.Engl.J.Med. 2002;346:393-403.

47.   Bhopal R, Fischbacher CM. Many South Asian people probably need pre-diabetes care. BMJ 2002;325:965.

48.   Cappuccio FP, Oakeshott P, Strazzullo P,Kerry SM Application of Framingham risk estimates to ethnic minorities in United Kingdom and implications for primary prevention of heart disease in general practice: cross sectional population based study BMJ 2002; 325: 1271.

4

Endothelial Dysfunction : Underlying mechanisms and their relevance for coronary heart disease in South Asians

A M Shah and M T Kearney

Introduction

The endothelial cell lining of the vasculature plays a fundamental role in maintaining vascular homeostasis in health, through multiple actions including the release of bioactive molecules (e.g. nitric oxide and prostacyclin) and the expression of surface molecules (e.g. tissue plasminogen activator (tPA)) and enzymatic activities (e.g., angiotensin converting enzyme (ACE)). nitric oxide has multiple actions in the vasculature, including flow-dependent vasodilatation, inhibition of leukocyte and platelet adhesion and aggregation, anti-proliferative and anti-apoptotic activity, and the inhibition of vessel permeability, which collectively tend to be anti-atherosclerotic. Compelling evidence supports a role for endothelial cell dysfunction as a key early event in the pathophysiology of atherosclerosis[1]. The term endothelial dysfunction encompasses a range of potential abnormalities, among which abnormalities of nitric oxide bioactivity, increased production of reactive oxygen species and the increased expression of cell surface adhesion molecules have received particular attention. It is now well established that the production or bioactivity of nitric oxide is reduced in conditions that predispose to atherosclerosis such as hypercholesterolaemia, diabetes mellitus, and cigarette smoking[1]. Endothelial dysfunction is often demonstrable years before any clinical manifestation of CHD. Furthermore, recent studies have shown that the presence of either coronary vascular or forearm vascular endothelial dysfunction in subjects without evidence of CHD is a powerful predictor of future major cardiovascular events [2,3].

CHD in UK South Asians

As discussed in chapter 1 by Bhopal, South Asian males have a greater CHD mortality than their white European counterparts[4]. Conventional risk factors alone do not account for the increased rates of CHD. Two potential reasons for the increased CHD rates in South Asians are an increased incidence of novel risk factors and/or an increased sensitivity to conventional risk factors (ie, an altered "dose-response" relationship). Environmental as well as genetic factors may be relevant to both these possibilities (Figure 4.1).

Figure 4.1. Potential reasons for increased incidence of atherosclerotic disease in South Asians

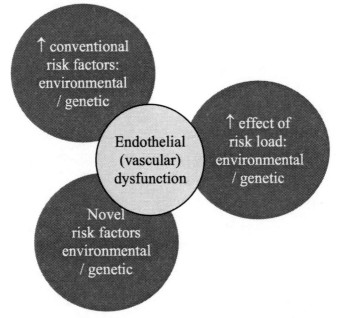

Although the evidence is not clear cut, as pointed out by Cruickshank *et al* in chapter 3, a higher prevalence of the metabolic syndrome (in particular the components of glucose intolerance and hyperinsulinaemia) may account for some of the excess CHD rates in South Asians[5,6]. Consonant with this, it has been shown that South Asian males are more insulin resistant than age-matched white European males, independent of generalised or truncal obesity[7]. Some of the reasons for the increased prevalence of insulin resistance may include reduced levels of physical activity and possibly amplified metabolic responses to particular diets, e.g. those high in carbohydrates[8]. For example, it has been shown that plasma insulin levels correlate closely with carbohydrate intake in South Asians[9].

An increased "dose-response" relationship to insulin resistance is suggested by findings such as the observation that South Asians with diabetes have CHD mortality rates higher than matched white European diabetics[10]. These data raise the intriguing possibility that the vasculature of South Asians and in particular younger South Asian males may be more susceptible to atherosclerosis when faced with components of the insulin resistance syndrome. In keeping with this, epidemiological studies looking at the relationship between carotid intima-media thickness and CHD prevalence in different ethnic populations have also suggested the possibility of a steeper "risk load-response" relationship in South Asians[11].

The link between insulin resistance, endothelial dysfunction and atherosclerosis

Insulin resistance is defined as resistance to the glucoregulatory actions of insulin. The underlying abnormality is thought to lie at one or more sites along the pathway linking the insulin receptor on the cell membrane to stimulation of glucose uptake *via* insulin-sensitive GLUT-4 membrane glucose transporters in the cell membrane[12]. A fundamental consequence of insulin resistance is fasting and postprandial hyperinsulinaemia, one effect of which is to stimulate hepatic triglyceride release. Resistance to the antilipolytic action of insulin increases the flux of non-esterified fatty acids (NEFAs), which augments the rise in triglyceride levels. Elevation of triglycerides and NEFAs are thus additional hallmarks of insulin resistance. NEFAs may further aggravate insulin resistance because of their effect to inhibit both glucose transport and key enzymes of glucose metabolism in skeletal muscle[13].

Hyperinsulinaemia, a contested risk factor *per se*, has been demonstrated to be an independent risk factor for the development of CHD, the magnitude of risk being of the same order as that of the well established risk factor of hypercholesterolaemia[14,15]. The IRAS study group demonstrated that insulin sensitivity is inversely proportional to the extent of atherosclerosis[16].

It is well established that the natural history of type 2 diabetes is often an insidious progression from insulin resistance with normoglycaemia to pancreatic decompensation and loss of glucose homeostasis. It is also likely that vascular disease in type 2 diabetes occurs before the onset of hyperglycaemia[17].

At least part of the increased atherogenic risk associated with insulin resistance may involve the development of endothelial dysfunction. Insulin resistance is associated with vascular endothelial dysfunction in humans[18], and there is a close correlation between insulin sensitivity and basal nitric oxide production in healthy subjects[19]. Insulin resistant non-diabetic relatives of patients with type 2 diabetes have impaired flow-dependent vasodilator responses (a surrogate marker of endothelial dysfunction), implying a reduction in nitric oxide bioavailability[20]. Flow-mediated vasodilation is also impaired in young South Asian males in comparison to age-matched white Europeans, independent of body mass index, cholesterol and HDL levels[21]. Evidence from animal studies also supports a causal relationship between insulin resistance and endothelial dysfunction[22].

Another aspect of endothelial function that may be implicated in the increased atherosclerotic risk associated with insulin resistance is the expression of adhesion molecules such as VCAM-1 and ICAM-1. Circulating levels of these adhesion molecules have a close and independent correlation with insulin resistance in healthy subjects[23]. Furthermore, recent evidence suggests that CRP, the concentration of which is inversely proportional to insulin sensitivity[24], is an independent risk factor for the development of atherosclerosis. This may involve the stimulation of adhesion molecule expression by vascular endothelial cells. Interestingly, C-reactive protein (CRP) has been shown to have several direct effects on endothelial cells including changes in nitric oxide synthase expression level.

Potential mechanisms underlying the relationship between insulin resistance and impaired NO bioactivity

Endothelial nitric oxide is generated from the amino acid L-arginine by the endothelial nitric oxide synthase enzyme (eNOS) in a reaction which requires tetrahydrobiopterin (BH_4) as a co-factor[1]. In general, a reduced bioactivity of endothelium-derived nitric oxide results from a reduced expression of eNOS, reduced activation of eNOS and/or the increased inactivation of nitric oxide by reactive oxygen species. The balance between nitric oxide production, reactive oxygen species production and antioxidant balance is increasingly recognized as key to endothelial homeostasis. Indeed, in subjects with endothelial dysfunction, a recent study showed that the presence of oxidative stress was a powerful independent predictor of future cardiovascular events[3]. In patients at high risk of developing CHD, a reduction in nitric oxide bioactivity is easily demonstrable *in vivo*, for example by impaired flow-mediated endothelial-dependent vasodilatation in the forearm or coronary vascular beds. Recent advances in endothelial biology indicate that these two responses reflect different subcellular mechanisms of eNOS activation and, importantly, may be differentially affected by insulin resistance. Whereas eNOS activation by agonists such as acetylcholine is calcium (Ca^{2+}) dependent, its sustained activation by shear stress involves the activation of PI3-kinase and then protein kinase B (or Akt) which causes eNOS phosphorylation[25,26]. The latter increases eNOS activity and its sensitivity to Ca^{2+}, so that it becomes active at subphysiological Ca^{2+} concentrations. Interestingly, the 'PI3-kinase / Akt pathway' is one of the primary subcellular pathways activated by insulin in many cell types, and has been shown to malfunction in cases of insulin resistance[12]. Furthermore, insulin is a vasodilator[27] that acts at least in part *via* the activation of PI3-kinase and Akt, leading to endothelial nitric oxide release[28]. An abnormality of the PI3-kinase / Akt pathway in the endothelium of insulin resistant subjects could therefore potentially contribute to endothelial dysfunction, particularly in response to increased blood flow or shear stress. Indeed, the vasodilator effect of insulin is blunted in insulin resistant humans[29]. Likewise, there is selective impairment of PI3-kinase-dependent Akt phosphorylation in isolated vessels of insulin resistant rats[30].

.

There is also evidence for the alternative mechanism of endothelial dysfunction, namely increased reactive oxygen species production, in insulin resistant states both experimentally and in patients. Recent studies indicate that major sources of reactive oxygen species that may contribute to endothelial dysfunction include dysfunctional nitric oxide synthases and phagocyte-type NADPH oxidases, both enzymes that can be regulated by pathophysiological stimuli implicated in the metabolic syndrome [1,31,32].

The role of obesity

Obesity increases the risk of developing cardiovascular atherosclerosis[33] and South Asians are known to have high rates of visceral adiposity relative to overall BMI as discussed in earlier chapters. The association between obesity and endothelial dysfunction is well established, both in animal studies and in man[34]. While a significant component of the increased risk associated with obesity may be related to the presence of insulin resistance, recent data indicate the additional possibility of alternative mechanisms. In particular, it has become evident that the adipocyte is not simply a fat storage cell but also an endocrine organ that releases bioactive proteins ("adipokines") in response to specific extracellular stimuli or perturbations in metabolic status. These adipokines include leptin, TNF-α and angiotensin II, all of which may potentially influence endothelial function and promote atherogenesis. Indeed, plasma levels of these adipokines are well established as being significantly elevated in obese humans. Thus, detailed studies here are also required to establish the influence of obesity on atherogenic risk independent of insulin resistance.

Conclusions

The thesis advanced in this article is that the increased risk of CHD in UK South Asians may be related both to a higher prevalence of metabolic dysregulation (insulin resistance and visceral obesity) and to an increased impact of the metabolic syndrome on the vasculature. Central to the ways in which metabolic dysregulation leads to atherosclerosis may be the role of endothelial dysfunction and activation. Investigation of the mechanistic relationship between insulin resistance, obesity, vascular dysfunction and atherosclerosis, both in white Europeans and South Asians, will be valuable in defining the basis for the increased CHD rates in South Asians and providing novel therapeutic targets. In addition, the reasons for the increased prevalence of metabolic syndrome *per se* in South Asians require elucidation. Both genetic and environmental influences are likely to be involved in these relationships.

Acknowledgements

The authors work in this field is supported by the British Heart Foundation. AMS holds the BHF Chair of Cardiology at King's College London. MTK is supported by a BHF Intermediate Fellowship award.

References

1. Cai H, Harrison DG. Endothelial dysfunction in cardiovascular diseases. The role of oxidant stress. Circ Res. 2000;87:840-844.

2. Schächinger V, Britten MB, Zeiher AM. Prognostic impact of coronary vasodilator dysfunction on adverse long-term outcome of coronary heart disease Circulation. 2000;101:1899–1906.

3. Heitzer T, Schlinzig T, Krohn K, Meinertz T, Münzel T. Endothelial dysfunction, oxidative stress, and risk of cardiovascular events in patients with coronary artery disease Circulation. 2001;104:2673-2678.

4. Balarajan R. Ethnicity and variations in mortality from coronary heart disease. Health Trends. 1996;28:45-51.

5. McKiegue PM, Ferrie JE, Pierpoint T, Marmot MG. Association of early-onset coronary heart disease in South Asian men with glucose intolerance and hyperinsulinaemia. Circulation. 1993;87:152-161.

6. McKeigue PM, Shah B, Marmot MG. Relation of central obesity and insulin resistance with high diabetes prevalence and cardiovascular risk in South Asians. Lancet. 1991;337:382-386.

7. Chandalia M, Abate N, Garg A, Stray-Gundersen J, Grundy SM. Relationship between generalised and upper body obesity to insulin resistance in Asian Indian men. J Clin Endocrinol Metab. 1999;84:2329-2335.

8. Coulston AM, Liu GC, Reaven GM. Plasma glucose, insulin and lipid responses to high-carbohydrate low-fat diets in normal humans. Metabolism. 1983;32:52-56.

9. Seevak L, McKeigue PM, Marmot MG. Relationship of hyperinsulinaemia to dietary intake in South Asian and European men. Am J Clin Nutr. 1994;59:1069-1074.

10. Chaturvedi N, Fuller J. Ethnic differences in the mortality from cardiovascular disease in the UK-do they persist in people with diabetes? J Epidemiol Comm Health. 1996;50:137-139.

11. Anand SS, Yusuf S, Vuksan V, et al. Differences in risk factors, atherosclerosis, and cardiovascular disease between ethnic groups in Canada: the Study of Health Assessment and Risk in Ethnic groups (SHARE). Lancet. 2000;356:279-284.

12. Shepherd PR, Kahn BB. Glucose transporters and insulin action – Implications for insulin resistance and diabetes mellitus. N Eng J Med. 1999;341:248-257.

13. Roden M, Price TB, Perseghin G, et al. Mechanism of free fatty acid-induced insulin resistance in humans. J Clin Invest. 1996;97:2859-2865.

14.   Despres JP, Lamarche B, Mauriege P, et al. Hyperinsulinaemia as an independent risk factor for ischaemic heart disease. N Eng J Med. 1996;334:952-957.

15.   Pyorala M, Miettinen H, Laakso M, Pyorala K. Hyperinsulinaemia predicts coronary heart disease risk in healthy middle aged men. The 22-year follow up results of the Helsinki policeman study. Circulation. 1998;98:398-404.

16.   Howard G, O'Leary DH, Zaccaro D, et al for the IRAS Investigators. Insulin sensitivity and atherosclerosis. Circulation. 1996;93:1809-1817.

17.   Haffner SM, Mykkanen L, Festa A, Burke JP, Stern MP. Insulin-resistant prediabetic subjects have more atherogenic risk factors than insulin-sensitive prediabetic subjects: implications for preventing coronary heart disease during the prediabetic state. Circulation. 2000;101:975-980.

18.   Steinberg HO, Chaker H, Leaming R, et al. Obesity/insulin resistance is associated with endothelial dysfunction. Implications for the syndrome of insulin resistance. J Clin Invest. 1996;97:2601-2610.

19.   Petrie JR, Ueda S, Webb DJ, Elliot HL, Connell JMC. Endothelial nitric oxide production and insulin sensitivity Circulation. 1996;93:1331-1333.

20.   Balletshofer BM, Rittig K, Enderle MD, et al. Endothelial dysfunction is detectable in young normotensive first-degree relatives of subjects with type 2 diabetes in association with insulin resistance. Circulation. 2000;101:1780-1784.

21.   Chambers JC, McGregor A, Jean-Marie J, Kooner JS. Abnormalities of vascular endothelial function may contribute to increased coronary heart disease risk in UK Indian Asians. Heart. 1999;81:501-504.

22.   Abe H, Yamada N, Kamata K, et al. Hypertension, hypertryglyceridaemia, and impaired endothelium-dependent vascular relaxation in mice lacking insulin receptor substrate-1. J Clin Invest. 1998;101:1784-1788.

23.   Chen NG, Holmes M, Reaven G. Relationship between insulin resistance, soluble adhesion molecules, and mononuclear cell binding in healthy volunteers. J Clin Endocrinol Metab. 1999;84:3485-3489.

24.   Yudkin JS, Stehouwer CDA, Emeis JJ, Coppack SW. C-reactive protein in healthy subjects: associations with obesity, insulin resistance and endothelial dysfunction. A potential role for cytokines originating from the adipose tissue. Arterioscler Thromb Vasc Biol. 1999;19:972-978.

25.   Dimmeler S, Fleming I, Fisslthaler B, et al. Activation of nitric oxide synthase in endothelial cells by Akt-dependent phosphorylation. Nature. 1999;399:601-605.

26.   Fulton D, Gratton J-P, McCabe TJ, et al. Regulation of endothelium derived nitric oxide production by the protein kinase Akt. Nature. 1999;399:597-601.

27.   Kearney MT, Cowley AJ, Evans A, Stubbs TA, Macdonald IA. Insulin's vasodepressor action on skeletal muscle vasculature: a novel mechanism for postprandial hypotension in the elderly. J Am Coll Cardiol. 1998;31:209-217.

28.   Zeng G, Quon MJ. Insulin-stimulated production of nitric oxide is inhibited by wortmannin. Direct measurement in vascular endothelial cells. J Clin Invest. 1996;98:894-898.

29.   Laakso M, Edelmen SV, Bretchel G, Baron AD. Decreased effect of insulin to stimulate skeletal muscle blood flow in obese man: a novel mechanism for insulin resistance. J Clin Invest. 1990;85:1844-1852.

30.   Jiang ZY, Lin Y-W, Clemont A, et al. Characterisation of selective insulin signaling in the vasculature of obese Zucker (fa/fa) rats. J Clin Invest. 1999;104:447-457.

31.   Li J-M, Shah AM. Mechanism of endothelial cell NADPH oxidase activation by angiotensin II: Role of the p47^{phox} subunit. J Biol Chem. 2003; (published Jan 30, 2003 as 10.1074/jbc.M209793200 at http://www.jbc.org/).

32.   Guzik TJ, Mussa S, Gastaldi D, et al. Mechanisms of increased vascular superoxide production in human diabetes mellitus: role of NAD(P)H oxidase and endothelial nitric oxide synthase. Circulation. 2002;105:1656-1662.

33.   Hubert B, Feinleib M, McNamara PM, Castelli WP. Obesity as an independent risk factor for cardiovascular disease: a 26- year follow-up of participants in the Framingham Heart Study. Circulation. 1983;67:968-977.

34.   Williams IL, Wheatcroft SB, Shah AM, Kearney MT. Obesity, atherosclerosis and the vascular endothelium: mechanisms of reduced nitric oxide bioavailability in humans. Int J Obesity. 2002;26:754-764.

5

Fetal and early life origins of cardiovascular disease in South Asians

C Fall

Introduction - the fetal origins hypothesis

Studies based on the follow-up of men and women whose birth weights were recorded have shown that poor fetal growth, indicated by a low weight at birth, is associated with an increased risk of adult cardiovascular disease (CVD). Some classical risk factors for CVD, including the metabolic syndrome and its component features - hypertension, type 2 diabetes, insulin resistance, truncal obesity, and dyslipidaemia also show associations with low birthweight. The fetal origins of adult disease (FOAD) hypothesis proposes that these reflect 'programming', whereby transient events, in this case fetal undernutrition, occurring at critical stages of development, have long-term effects on the body's structure and function[1]. Fetal adaptations to undernutrition, to conserve nutrients and prioritise brain growth, include reduced secretion of and sensitivity to the fetal growth hormones insulin and IGF-I (insulin like growth factor –type 1), altered body composition (reduced muscle growth), and impaired development of some abdominal organs (reduced renal nephron numbers and pancreatic beta cells). The glucocorticoid system is up-regulated. According to the FOAD hypothesis these changes have permanent metabolic effects that lead to later disease. An alternative hypothesis is that both low birth weight and adult disease have common genetic antecedents.

The effects of low birthweight on later CVD risk are modified by the pattern of post-natal growth. Although greater weight gain in infancy (the first 12 post-natal months) is associated with a reduced CVD risk, the reverse is true for weight gain (and fat gain) during childhood, adolescence and adult life, all of which are associated with an increased risk. Childhood and adult BMI interact with size at birth. The adverse effects of obesity on cardiovascular risk are greatest in people who were small at birth[2]. The effects of this mis-match between fetal 'thrift' and post-natal 'plenty' has been called 'adaptation-dysadaptation'.

Recent studies indicate that in addition to the adverse effects of low birthweight, there are problems at very high birthweights. Offspring of mothers with gestational diabetes, which causes fetal overnutrition (macrosomia) have an increased risk of obesity and type 2 diabetes compared with offspring of non-diabetic mothers or women who became diabetic after the pregnancy. There is therefore a U-shaped or J-shaped relationship between birthweight and adult type 2 diabetes, with increased rates of disease at both low and very high birthweights[3].

An explanation for CVD in South Asians?

Poor fetal growth may contribute to the current epidemic of CVD occurring in South Asian populations. CVD in South Asians is often associated with insulin resistance and the metabolic syndrome, the risk factors which have been consistently linked with low birthweight. Mean birthweight in the Indian subcontinent is 2.6-2.8 kg, the lowest in the world, and remains low in UK South Asians. Poor weight gain in infancy is also common. At the same time, recent improvements in nutrition, resulting from urbanisation or migration abroad, enable small babies to catch-up. Both childhood and adolescent obesity are rapidly emerging problems. Increasing numbers of South Asians are therefore making the 'high-risk' journey from intrauterine nutritional poverty to post-natal nutritional affluence. There are few data from India on the prevalence of gestational diabetes, but studies of South Asian migrants to the UK and elsewhere have shown rates of gestational diabetes approximately 5 times those of the white European population.

FOAD research in India

Studies designed to test the FOAD hypothesis have been carried out in India at the KEM Hospital, Pune (children) and Holdsworth Memorial Hospital, Mysore (adults) using birth data recorded in obstetric notes. In Pune, low birthweight children (at 8 years) had increased blood pressure, LDL-cholesterol concentrations and subscapular/triceps skinfold ratios[4], and those with a high childhood weight and fat mass also had raised plasma insulin (Figure 5.1) and IGF-I concentrations and urinary glucocorticoid excretion. In Mysore, among 20-40 year old adults, lower birthweight was associated with impaired glucose tolerance, higher plasma insulin and triglyceride concentrations and ischaemic ECG changes[5]. Among older adults (40-60 years), there were associations between low birthweight and clinical coronary heart disease and insulin resistance (Figure 5.2)[6,7]. In this older age group the findings for type 2 diabetes differed from the younger men and women. Diabetes occurred more commonly in those who were heavy relative to their length at birth (high ponderal index, birthweight/length[3]), and whose mothers were heaviest during pregnancy[7]. This may reflect gestational diabetes.

Determinants of low birthweight in South Asians

Size at birth is determined by both genes and environment. The mother's nutritional status is one of the most important modifiable factors. Nutrition throughout the life cycle of a female influences the fetal growth of her offspring. Studies of contemporary pregnancies in Pune and Mysore showed that the mother's fat mass (a measure of her current nutrition), her height and head circumference (her childhood growth) and her birthweight (her own fetal growth) all predicted the birthweight of her offspring[8]. Genetic effects, indicated by correlations between paternal size and offspring birthweight were significant, but weaker than maternal effects, and related mainly to fetal skeletal growth (length and head size). In the Indian neonates, non-fat soft tissues (muscle and abdominal circumference) were reduced by about two standard deviation scores compared with UK white European babies, but body fat (skinfold thickness) was relatively preserved[9]. The well-known propensity of South Asian populations for central obesity thus appears to be present at birth. Neonatal body fat correlated with the mother's body fat, plasma glucose and triglyceride concentrations.

Neonatal size was also related to maternal diet. In a rural area near Pune (the Pune Maternal Nutrition Study) mothers with higher intakes of green leafy vegetables (GLVs), fruit and milk and higher red cell folate and plasma vitamin C concentrations had babies that were larger in all measurements at birth[10]. Birth size was not related to

Figure 5.1. Relative insulin resistance (RIR-HOMA) in 8 year old children of Pune, India.

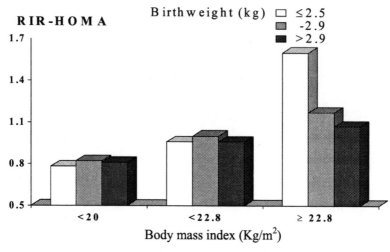

Bavdekar et al. Diabetes 2000;48:2422-2429

Figure 5.2. Relative insulin resistance (RIR-HOMA) in 40-60 year old men, Mysore, India.

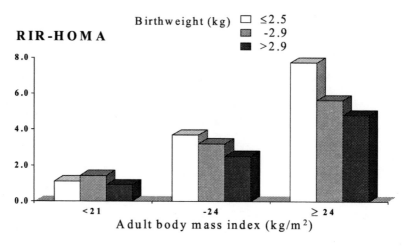

Fall et al. Diabetic Med 1998;15:220

maternal energy or protein intakes. These data suggest that micronutrients, for which GLVs, fruit and milk are rich sources, may be important limiting factors for fetal growth in this undernourished population (mean maternal BMI 18 kg/m^2). This is currently being tested in a food supplementation study in Mumbai. Another factor in the rural population was maternal physical workload. Mothers with higher energy expenditure, determined using a workload questionnaire, had smaller babies[11]. There were striking associations between the most strenuous activities, such as carrying water from the well, and hand-washing clothes, and lower birthweight. The factors responsible for persisting low birthweights among UK South Asians must be quite different; however, effects of the mother's own fetal experience on her capacity to nourish her fetus may lead to a delay of at least one generation before nutritional improvements in any population lead to substantial gains in fetal growth.

The prevalence of gestational diabetes was low (0.2%) in the rural Pune population, but high (6%) among urban mothers in Mysore[12]. The relative adiposity of the Indian neonate was exaggerated further in babies of diabetic mothers. Future studies are under way to examine effects of maternal diet and gestational diabetes, and childhood growth patterns, on the development of CVD risk.

Two new cohort studies of young adults in New Delhi and Vellore, are currently taking place, funded by the British Heart Foundation. Numbering around 2,000 in each centre these unique cohorts have exceptionally detailed data from before pregnancy (maternal and paternal height and weight), at birth (birthweight, birth length, head circumference, accurate gestational age) and throughout childhood (weight, height and head size during infancy, childhood and adolescence). A range of CVD risk factors are being measured and these studies will be particularly helpful in determining how post-natal growth affects the risk of adult disease.

Implications for prevention of disease and future research

Cardiovascular disease and type 2 diabetes have reached 'epidemic' proportions in South Asian populations. If fetal nutrition is an important factor in their aetiology, preventive measures will need to focus on improvements in fetal growth and development, as well as on adult lifestyles. Better nutrition of girls and of young women before and during pregnancy are obvious recommendations for South Asian populations still suffering from overt undernutrition. It is not clear, however, how to improve fetal development in mothers who may have experienced undernutrition in their own fetal life and childhood, and who are stunted, but who are well-nourished as adult women. Indeed there are risks if they become overnourished; they should certainly avoid frank obesity, which carries an increased risk of gestational diabetes, and increases body fat in the fetus. More research is needed into the effects of the mother's dietary quality on fetal growth. While few women in the UK are lacking sufficient dietary energy and protein, their micronutrient status is often less than ideal, especially in lower income families who cannot afford fresh vegetables and dairy products. This is true in all ethnic groups, not just South Asians.

Avoidance of obesity in childhood is important for many reasons and in all ethnic groups. The imperative is probably even greater for South Asian children. The relative adiposity of South Asians means that at any level of BMI, they have a higher fat mass than other ethnic groups. Increased risk for later disease starts at lower levels of BMI, indeed at BMI levels which would not be considered obese by UK standards. These risks are greater still for the individual who started out as small-for-dates babies. Type 2 diabetes, previously considered an adult disease, is already appearing among children in the UK, especially South Asian children. Prevention of childhood obesity, and promotion of physical activity in children, needs to go out as a very strong public health message, and as a matter of urgency, to South Asian families.

Opportunities to study fetal and early life determinants of CVD in UK South Asians are limited by a paucity of good quality longitudinal data for mothers, neonates and children. There is a need for birth cohorts from all ethnic groups to be established and prospectively followed up in the UK.

Acknowledgements

With thanks to colleagues in India, especially Anand Pandit and Chittaranjan Yajnik, KEM Hospital, Pune; Shobha Rao, Agharkar Research Institute, Pune; and SR Veena and Prasad Karat, Holdsworth Memorial Hospital, Mysore. The research has been funded by the Wellcome Trust, the British Heart Foundation, the Parthenon Trust,

DFID, the Wessex Medical Trust, and the MRC. I also thank Sneha India (www.sneha-india.org) for its support.

References

1. Barker DJP Mothers, babies and health in later life. Churchill Livingstone, London 1994.

2. Eriksson JG, Forsen T, Tuomilehto J, Winter PD, Osmond C, Barker DJP. Catch-up growth in childhood and death from coronary heart disease: longitudinal study. BMJ 1999;318, 427-31.

3. Rich-Edwards JW, Colditz GA, Stampfer MJ, Willett WC, Gillman MW, Hennekens CH, Speizer F, Mason J. Birthweight and the risk of type 2 diabetes in adult women. Ann Int Med 1999;130:278-84.

4. Bavdekar A, Yajnik CS, Fall CHD, Bapat S, Pandit AN, Deshpande V, Bhave S, Kellingray SD, Joglekar C. The insulin resistance syndrome (IRS) in eight-year-old Indian children: small at birth, big at 8 years or both? Diabetes 2000;48:2422-9.

5. Fall CHD. Developing Countries and Affluence in Type 2 Diabetes: the thrifty phenotype. Ed DJP Barker. British Medical Bulletin 2001;60:33-50.

6. Stein C, Fall CHD, Kumaran K, Osmond C, Cox V, Barker DJP. Fetal growth and coronary heart disease in South India. Lancet 1996;348:1269-73.

7. Fall CHD, Stein C, Kumaran K, Cox V, Osmond C, Barker DJP, Hales CN. Size at birth, maternal weight, and non-insulin-dependent diabetes (NIDDM) in South Indian adults. Diabetic Medicine 1998;15:220-7.

8. Fall CHD, Yajnik CS, Rao S, Coyaji KJ, Shier RP. The effects of maternal body composition before birth on fetal growth: the Pune Maternal nutrition and Fetal Growth Study. In: eds. O'Brien PMS, Wheeler T, Barker DJP. Fetal Programming; Influences on development and disease in later life. RCOG Press, London, 1999.

9. Yajnik CS, Fall CHD, Coyaji KJ, Hirve SS, Rao S, Barker DJP, Joglekar C, Kellingray S. Neonatal anthropometry: the thin-fat Indian baby; the Pune Maternal Nutrition Study. Int J Obesity 2003;27:173-80.

10. Rao S, Yajnik CS, Kanade A, Fall CHD, Margetts BM, Jackson AA, Shier R, Joshi S, Rege S, Lubree H, Desai B. Maternal fat intakes and micronutrient status are related to fetal size at birth in rural India; the Pune Maternal Nutrition Study. J Nutr 2001;131:1217-1224.

11.   Rao S, Kanade A, Margetts BM, Yajnik CS, Lubree H, Rege S, Desai B, Jackson AA, Fall CHD. Maternal activity in relation to birth size in rural India; the Pune Maternal Nutrition Study. Eur J Clin Nutr 2003 (in press).

12.   Hill JC, Krishnaveni GV, Fall CHD, Kellingray SD. Glucose tolerance and insulin status during pregnancy in South India: relationships to maternal and neonatal body composition. J Endocrinol 2000;164 (Suppl): P252.

6

Coronary heart disease in South Asian populations - the role of genetics

NJ Samani and P Sharma

Introduction

As discussed previously, the only logical explanation to account for the increase in CHD in South Asians arising from urbanization or migration is that it is a reaction to an adverse environment. Clearly, given the short time span involved in the emergence of the epidemic, genetic factors cannot solely be responsible and this has led to a minimization of their importance in most reviews. We propose here that elucidation of the genetic factors that predispose to CHD in South Asians is central to a fuller understanding of the epidemic and the nature of gene-environment interactions in the aetiology of CHD. Given this potential, we highlight the paucity of studies on genetics of CHD in South Asians and the relative lack of inclusion of South Asians in ongoing or planned genetic epidemiological studies and discuss the reasons behind this. We highlight the urgent need to address and rectify this deficit.

CHD has an important genetic contribution, especially in its more premature form. Thus, family studies in white European subjects have shown that a history of CHD before the age of 55 years in a 1st degree relative increases the risk in an individual by up to 10 fold[1]. This applies equally to subjects originating from South Asia. Francke et al[2] report a 7.4-fold increased prevalence in siblings of Mauritian Asians affected by CHD.

Another epidemiological observation that highlights the likely importance of genetic factors is the striking contrast in incidence of CHD in different ethnic groups e.g. higher rates of CHD in South Asians compared to Afro-Carribean and Chinese populations [3,4] (also see Table 1.1A in Introductory chapter by Bhopal). These differences cannot be fully accounted for by conventional risk factors alone and suggests a role for genetic factors in determining the prevalence of disease.

The last decade has seen significant efforts attempting to elucidate the genetic basis of CHD. The main approach used has been a case-control design[5] where the frequency of a candidate gene variant in subjects with a specified CHD phenotype is compared with those without such a phenotype. Variants in several genes involved in lipid metabolism, thrombosis and vascular biology have been associated with risk of myocardial infarction or other CHD phenotypes[6]. A major issue that has limited application of the data has been inconsistent replication of primary findings in subsequent studies[6]. Important contributory factors to this include the low power of many studies, varying definitions of the phenotype, genetic heterogeneity between the populations studied, and a likely major modulating impact of gene-environment interactions[5,6]. Nonetheless, a role for several gene variants now seems highly probable with similar findings across multiple studies, supported by findings in prospective studies and in "meta-analyses" [6]. More recently, results of family-based genetic approaches are beginning to emerge in the CHD field[2,7,8]. The most common approach that has been adopted has been the affected sib-pair approach where large numbers of families with more than one affected sibling are analysed using anonymous genetic markers to identify regions of the genome that are shared more commonly than by chance by the affected siblings[5]. These regions are thus likely to contain either a single gene or multiple genes that affect the risk of CHD in a proportion of the families. The advantages of the linkage approach are first, that there is no *a priori* assumption of the likely nature of the gene(s) involved and second that the whole genome can be screened. The disadvantages are that the studies need large number of individuals to obtain adequate power to detect modest effects and when linkages are identified there is a still considerable effort required to identify the causal gene and variant within the region[5]. The most persuasive example of this approach to date in CHD has been a mapping of a locus on chromosome 14 in 513 white European families which was associated with an increased risk of myocardial infarction[7]. Interestingly, one of the first genome-wide search for loci predisposing to CHD has been conducted in a South Asian origin population – Indo-Mauritians – who are known to have a prevalence of CHD which is amongst the highest in the world[2]. 99

independent families of North Eastern Indian origin were recruited for a genome scan using 403 microsatellite markers. The proband was required to be affected at a young age (<52 years) in an attempt to further enhance the genetic contribution to their disease. Suggestive linkage for CHD was obtained for regions on chromosome 16p13-pter and 10q23. This region partially overlapped with a linkage peak for hypertension.

Having provided a brief review of the genetic approaches to CHD, the main purpose of this paper is not to tabulate and review the few genetic studies that have been done on CHD in South Asians but to consider potential underlying genetic explanations for the increased incidence of CHD in South Asian subjects compared with other ethnic groups.

Theoretically, at least, there are 3 possibilities (Table 6.1). First, that there are gene variants that are specific and exclusive to South Asians that increase their risk. There is little epidemiological or genetic evidence to support this so this explanation seems unlikely. Second, certain risk alleles may be more prevalent in South Asians compared to other ethnic groups. These variations in prevalence may be due to chance or more likely a consequence of evolutionary advantage that they provided at some stage in the divergence of ethnic groups. The "thrifty gene" hypothesis initially proposed by James van Gundia Neel falls into this category[9]. Simply put, this much-debated hypothesis proposes that there are genetic variants that were protective and enhanced survival at a time when calories and salt were less abundant, but harmful in the presence of increased caloric intake[9]. Such alleles could be more common in South Asians and predispose to central obesity and diabetes mellitus, which are important predisposing factors for CHD in these subjects[10]. Interestingly, Davey and colleagues[11] have shown that central fat distribution is highly heritable in South Asian families. In trying to identify genetic variants that may underlie the "thrifty gene" hypothesis the focus has rightly been on genes and pathways involved in the insulin resistance metabolic syndrome[12] (also see Chapter 2). However, the nature of the genetic pathways remain unclear. There is emerging evidence that functional or function-associated variants in other cardiovascular genes show significant inter-ethnic variations. For example, the D allele of the angiotensin converting enzyme (ACE), which is associated with higher plasma ACE levels is less common in South Asians subjects then in white Europeans or people of African origin[13].

Lipoprotein(a) (Lp[a]) is another genetically- determined risk factor for CHD, especially when accompanied by increased concentrations of LDL [14]. Some studies have shown that South Asians have higher plasma levels of Lp[a], whether living in the United Kingdom or in Punjab, compared to white European subjects[15], presumably due to a higher prevalence of variants in the apolipoprotein (a) gene that increase Lp[a][14]. The capacity of a migrating population to rapidly acquire a raised LDL cholesterol level due to changes in dietary patterns and/or life-style shows how a genetically determined CHD risk factor – increased Lp[a] – can be transformed into a more potent risk factor by westernization[16]. This example emphasises the importance of considering the role of genetics if we are to fully understand the epidemic of CHD in South Asians. It illustrates, the concept of gene-environment interactions (the third of the possible scenarios illustrated in Table 6.1), which must ultimately determine CHD risk. It is important to recognise that variation in risk may occur where the frequency of disease associated alleles is similar in different ethnic groups but the exposure to the relevant environmental risk factor varies. Possible environmental risk factors that may differ between ethnic groups include those related to diet, physical activity, smoking and those that are less easy to quantify such as stress. The point is that emphasising either environmental factors or genetic factors alone produces an incomplete picture.

We propose that identifying differences in inter-ethnic prevalence of functional variants in key cardiovascular system (CVS) pathways and understanding their impact on intermediary phenotypes in particular environmental settings provides a powerful and efficient strategy to dissecting the genetic basis of complex traits (Figure 6.1).

Table 6.1. Possible genetic explanations for increased risk of coronary heart disease in South Asians

1. Disease-related mutations specific to South Asian populations
2. Increased prevalence of susceptibility alleles
3. Adverse gene-environment interactions

Figure 6.1: Use of inter-ethnic differences in functional genetic variants to dissect the genetic basis of coronary heart disease

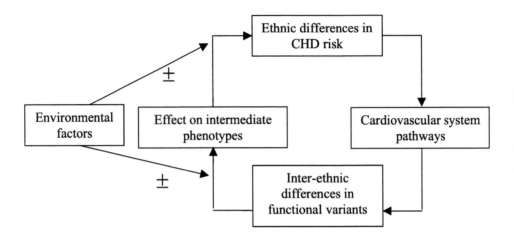

Given this potential, it is noteworthy that few genetic studies in CHD have been done in subjects of South Asian origin and indeed many of the large genetic projects in Western counties have specifically excluded non-white subjects[17]. Although the immediate rationale for this is understandable, namely to optimise power and try and minimize genetic heterogeneity and population stratification as a cause of misleading (false positive) findings[5], future projects need to consider the gains to be had, especially in studies focusing on functional variants and intermediary biochemical or physiological phenotypes on the causal pathway to disease. However, even where participation is open to all communities, uptake by ethnic minority groups and particularly South Asian groups is low. For example, in the BHF Family Heart Study, less than 2% of the over 2000 families recruited come from a South Asian background despite a concentration of recruitment effort in areas with large South Asian communities (NJ Samani, unpublished data). The reasons behind the low participation of ethnic minority groups in genetic studies need to be identified and addressed. The information provided may be insensitive to issues of culture and religion, as well as language. Benefits of participation may not be clear. In addition, the word 'genetic' may have perceived consequences to families with regard to stigma within a relatively closed community. Whether some of these factors could be overcome by better and more culturally specific information sensitive to religious concerns requires to be investigated. Especially, with major long-term projects such as UK Biobank[18] about to start, it is important that barriers to participation of ethnic minority groups in genetic research are overcome so that we can fully gain from understanding the gene-environment interactions that underlie inter-ethnic variation in risk of CHD as well as other cardiovascular conditions.

Conclusion

Genetics plays an important role in the pathogenesis of CHD in South Asians as it does in other ethnic groups. The epidemic of CHD in South Asians as a consequence of migration and/or westernisation is likely to have its root in adverse gene-environment interactions. Elucidation of the genetic factors that predispose to CHD in South Asians is essential if we are to fully understand its nature and devise appropriate and specific strategies for its prevention and treatment.

Acknowledgments

NJS is a British Heart Foundation Professor of Cardiology.

References

1.   Marenberg ME, Risch N, Berkman LF, Floderus B, de Faire U. Genetic susceptibility to death from coronary heart disease in a study of twins. N Engl J Med 1988; 318:727-732.

2.   Francke S, Manraj M, Lacquemant C, Lecoeur C, Lepretre F, Passa P, Hebe A, Corset L, Yan SLK, Lahmidi S, Jankee S, Gunness TK, Ramjuttun US, Balgobin V, Dina C, Froguel P. A genome-wide scan for coronary heart disease suggests in Indo-Mauritians a susceptibility locus on chromosome 16p13 and replicates linkage with the metabolic syndrome. Hum Mol Genet 2001; 24:2751-2765.

3.   Chaturvedi N. Ethnic differences in cardiovascular disease. Heart 2003; 89:681-686.

4.   Wild S, McKeigue P. Cross sectional analysis of mortality by country of birth in England and Wales, 1970-92. BMJ 1997; 314:705-709.

5.   Lander ES, Schork NJ. Genetic dissection of complex traits. Science 1994; 265: 2037-2048.

6.   Samani NJ, Singh R. Molecular genetics of acute coronary syndromes. In: Current challenges in acute coronary syndromes. De Bono DP, Sobel E (eds). Blackwell Science, Oxford, 2001: 81-98.

7.   Broeckel U, Hengstenberg C, Mayer B, Holmer S, Martin LJ, Comuzzie AG, Blangero J, Nurnberg P, Reis A, Riegger GA, Jacob HJ, Schunkert H. A comprehensive linkage analysis for myocardial infarction and its related risk factors. Nature Genetics 2002; 30:210-214.

8.   Harrap SB, Zammit KS, Wong ZY, Williams FM, Bahlo M, Tonkin AM, Anderson ST. Genome-wide linkage analysis of the acute coronary syndrome suggests a locus on chromosome 2. Arterioscler Thromb Vasc Biol. 2002; 22:874-878.

9.   Neel JV, Weder AB, Julius S. Type II diabetes, essential hypertension, and obesity as "syndromes of impaired genetic homeostasis": the "thrifty genotype" hypothesis enters the 21st century. Perspect Biol Med. 1998; 42:44-74.

10.   MeKeigue PM, Shah B, Marmot MG. Relation of central obesity and insulin resistance with high diabetes prevalence and cardiovascular risk in South Asians. Lancet 1991; 337:382-386.

11.   Davey G, Ramachandran A, Snehalatha C, Hitman GA, McKeigue PM. Familial aggregation of central obesity in Southern Indians. Int J Obes Relat Metab Disord. 2000; 24:1523-1527.

12.   Groop L. Genetics of the metabolic syndrome. Br J Nutr 2000;83 Suppl 1:S39-S48.

13.   Sagnella GA, Rothwell MJ, Onipinla AK, Wicks PD, Cook DG, Cappuccio FP. A population study of ethnic variations in the angiotensin-converting enzyme I/D polymorphism: relationships with gender, hypertension and impaired glucose metabolism. J Hypertens 1999; 17:657-664.

14.   Editorial. Lipoprotein (a). Lancet 1991; 331:397-398.

15.   Bhatnagar D, Anand IS, Durrington PN, Patel DJ, Wander GS, Mackness MI, Creed F, Tomenson B, Chandrashekhar Y, Winterbotham M, Britt RP, Keil JE, Sutton GC. Coronary risk factors in people from the Indian subcontinent living in West London and their siblings in India. Lancet 1995; 345:405-409.

16.   Williams B. Westernised Asians and cardiovascular disease: nature or nurture? Lancet 1995; 345:410-402.

17.   Caulfield M, Munroe P, Pembroke J, Samani N, Dominiczak A, Brown M, Benjamin N, Webster J, Ratcliffe P, O'Shea S, Papp J, Taylor E, Dobson R, Knight J, Newhouse S, Hooper J, Lee W, Brain N, Clayton D, Lathrop GM, Farrall M, Connell J. MRC British Genetics of Hypertension Study. Genome-wide mapping of human loci for essential hypertension. Lancet 2003; 361:2118-2123.

18.   UK Biobank: http://www.ukbiobank.ac.uk.

7

Inflammation and infection in coronary heart disease - a role in South Asians?

S Gupta

Introduction

Coronary heart disease continues to be the commonest cause of death in the industrialised world and is ever-increasing in developing countries[1]. As discussed in earlier chapters, conventional risk factors for atherosclerosis and CHD (such as tobacco smoking, diabetes mellitus, hyperlipidaemia and hypertension) are well recognised but fail to fully account for the varying prevalence and severity of disease, in different populations[2]. A number of potential 'novel' atherogenic markers have been proposed in recent years; infection with common micro-organisms maybe one such risk factor which will be the focus in this chapter (Table 7.1)[3,4]. Atherosclerosis is an inflammatory disease[5]. At each stage through atherogenesis, mature lesion development, plaque rupture and presentation with acute clinical events, inflammation plays a pivotal role. Serum CRP, a non-specific marker of inflammation, has also been found to be closely associated with cardiovascular risk and subsequent events – and may be a potent marker in South Asians[6].

Whether antigens of infective micro-organisms are an additional 'signal' for the inflammation is an intriguing and feasible possibility – but as yet proven. Many micro-organisms have been associated with atherosclerosis (see table 7.1). *Chlamydia pneumoniae* has emerged as the most likely 'culprit' pathogen of all to have a causal role in atherosclerosis[4]. For this reason, this chapter focuses on this micro-organism, but the difficulties shown in demonstrating cause and effect are indicative of findings in other micro-organisms. It is a gram-negative, obligate intracellular pathogen, **Table 7.1. Micro-organisms implicated in atherosclerosis**

Micro-organism	Author and Year of Publication
Bacillus typhosus	1889, Gilbert and Lion
Streptococci	1931, Benson *et al*
Coxsackie B virus	1968, Sohal *et al*
Adenovirus	1973, Fabricant *et al*
Mycoplasma gallisepticum	1973, Clyde and Thomas
Marek's disease virus	1978, Fabricant *et al*
Cytomegalovirus	1987, Petrie *et al*
Herpes simplex virus	1987, Hajjar *et al*
Chlamydia pneumoniae	1988, Saikku *et al*
Measles virus	1990, Csonka *et al*
Epstein-Barr virus	1993, Straka *et al*
Human immunodeficiency virus	1993, Paton *et al*
Helicobacter pylori	1994, Mendall *et al*
Mycoplasma fermentans	1996, Ong *et al*
Coxiella burnetti	1999, Lovey *et al*
Porphyromonas gingivalis	1999, Chiu *et al*
Streptococcus sanguis	1999, Chiu *et al*
Actinobacillus actinomycetemcomitans	2000, Haraszthy *et al*
Bacteroides forsythus	2000, Haraszthy *et al*
Hepatitis A virus	2000, Zhu *et al*
Influenza virus	2000, Naghavi *et al*
Prevotella intermedia	2000, Haraszthy *et al*

primarily causing respiratory symptoms and complications in adults, and accounts for 5-20% of all cases of community acquired pneumonias[7]. Infection with *C. pneumoniae* is usually benign but is a global phenomenon – with a seroprevalence of

50-70% in middle aged and older adults, irrespective of social class and geographical population[8].

Chlamydia pneumoniae and atherosclerosis

The evidence implicating *C pneumoniae* in atherosclerosis could be subdivided into the following areas of investigation:

1. Seroepidemiological data
2. Direct identification of the micro-organism within plaque
3. Animal models showing induction or acceleration of atherosclerosis
4. Infection triggering pro-atherogenic and pro-thrombotic responses in various cells
5. Preliminary anti-*chlamydial* antibiotic studies in humans

Seroepidemiological data

Saikku *et al* in 1988 were the first to demonstrate that elevated serological markers of *C pneumoniae* infection were positively associated with CHD[9]. Since the original publication, some 80 subsequent studies worldwide have now been reported[10]. Furthermore, an association between antibodies to *C pneumoniae* and atherosclerosis in arterial sites (other than the coronary arteries) has also been reported[3]. Both positive and negative[11] correlations between increasing antibody titres and presence and severity of atherosclerotic disease have been published. The lack of a standardised microimmunofluorescence test, a variable cut-off titre defining seropositivity, and incomplete adjustment for confounding factors may explain the lack of correlation seen with the larger prospective antibody studies[12].

Plaque studies

In 1992, Shor *et al* first detected *C pneumoniae* in atherosclerotic lesions of the coronary arteries at an autopsy study[13]. More than 100 subsequent pathological specimen studies have since demonstrated *C pneumoniae* in a wide variety of arterial specimens, including occluded bypass grafts[3], using techniques of immunocytochemistry, polymerase chain reaction and electron microscopy. Overall, the detection rate of *C pneumoniae* is approximately 60% in atherosclerotic lesions, versus 3% in control (non-atherosclerotic) arterial specimens[3,14].

Chlamydia pneumoniae has also been identified in human non-cardiovascular tissue – such has lung, liver, spleen, bone marrow and lymph node – reflecting its ubiquitous presence[15]. The mere presence of the micro-organism in atherosclerotic lesions does not necessarily infer a direct pathogenetic role. The 'innocent bystander' hypothesis supports the notion that *C pneumoniae* could merely be carried by circulatory monocytes from the site of infection to remain dormant in various tissues. However a report by Jackson *et al* has shown that *C pneumoniae* detection rate was between 29-50% in cardiovascular tissue versus 5-13% in non-cardiovascular tissue[15]. Such findings could be interpreted as refuting the 'innocent bystander' notion. There are only a few reports of negative pathological specimen studies and the micro-organism is very rarely found in 'normal' segments of arterial specimens[16]. Perhaps to a greater significance live 'viable' micro-organisms can now be cultured from plaque[17,18] and this adds weight to a direct pathogenetic role.

Infection-induced atherosclerosis in animals
Elegant animal experiments in the 1970's demonstrated herpesvirus-induced atherogenesis[19]. Analogous to this, Fong *et al* and colleagues infected rabbits intranasally with *C pneumoniae*[20]. The animals developed atheromatous changes in the aortic wall. Cholesterol supplementation in such infected rabbits increases intimal thickening whilst lesion thickness has been shown to be less marked in infected rabbits given azithromycin, an antibiotic which is active against *C pneumoniae*[21]. Animal models have shown the pathogenetic role in terms of temporal sequence and infective dose of infection and subsequent development of lesions. To what extent the pathophysiology and 'acutely induced' atherogenesis (i.e. within weeks) in laboratory animals reflects chronic human atherosclerosis remains to be clarified.

Pro-thrombotic and pro-inflammatory mechanisms
Laboratory based studies have shown that *C pneumoniae* organisms infect and proliferate in cells such as macrophages, endothelial cells and smooth muscle cells, which form the main constituents of the atherosclerotic plaque[22-24]. Infection may contribute to endothelial dysfunction and lead to the expression of inflammatory markers such as fibrinogen, CRP, cytokines, chemokines and adhesion molecules[22]. Several of these markers are potential predictors for first and future cardiovascular events. *Chlamydia pneumoniae*, by being transported from the alveolar macrophage

via the circulating monocyte direct reaches the distant endothelial cell surface[25] (Table 7.2). Indeed, viable micro-organisms facilitate the preferential adhesion of infected monocytes to human coronary artery endothelial and smooth muscle cells.

Table 7.2. Pathophysiology of the link between inflammation, infection and atherosclerosis

Link between inflammation, infection and atherosclerosis
1. Replication within alveolar macrophages and dissemination within monocytes
2. Direct infection of coronary artery endothelium
3. Migrating monocytes carry organism to subendothelial layers
4. Macrophage activation leading to local inflammation
5. Cytokine release triggering endothelial damage
6. Enhanced procoagulant state
7. T-cell activation
8. Immune cross reactivity with heat shock proteins
9. Genetic susceptibility to infection

Recently *C pneumoniae* and *Chlamydial* heat shock protein (HSP)60 were shown to stimulate human vascular muscle cell proliferation and also activate macrophage TNF-alpha and matrix metalloproteinases enzymes (which contribute to connective tissue degradation and atherosclerotic plaque rupture[26]). That the *Chlamydial* HSP60 and human HSP60 frequently co-localise within atherosclerotic plaques, sheds light on an autoimmune process linking infection, inflammation and atherogenesis. In contrast to the humoral immunity to *C pneumoniae,* specific cell-mediated immunity in CHD has also been demonstrated. As an additional or independent mechanism *C pneumoniae* may induce a hypercoaguable state promoting atherothrombosis[27] and enhanced expression of adhesion molecules such, as VCAM and ICAM-1 (as discussed by Shah in chapter 4).

Antibiotic intervention studies in humans

Interest in human antibiotic trials in the context of *C pneumoniae* infection and atherosclerosis was triggered by the publication of two pilot clinical studies in 1997. In a UK-based study[28] survivors of myocardial infarction (MI) were screened for antibody levels for *C pneumoniae*. Increasing anti-*chlamydial* antibodies were associated with increasing adverse cardiovascular events. However, patients with elevated IgG antibodies, randomised to receive azithromycin, had a 5-fold reduction in events compared to those receiving placebo. Patients receiving azithromycin also had a greater change in serum and monocyte markers of activation and inflammation. In a similar Argentinean study[29], another macrolide, roxithromycin, given to patients with an acute coronary syndrome appeared to reduce adverse cardiac events at 30 days. Inflammatory markers such as CRP decreased more significantly in the roxithromycin-treated group. A series of studies examining the effects of antibiotic prescribing and cardiovascular events ensued. Results have been mixed. In a large case-control study comparing over 3,000 patients (with an index MI) to over 13,000 controls the cases of MI were significantly less likely to have been given quinolones or tetracyclines (i.e.anti-*chlamydial* antibiotics) in the preceding 3 years, compared to controls[30]. More recently, Pilote *et al* showed that exposure to antichlamydial antibiotics during the 3 months after acute MI was associated with a small survival benefit[31]. By contract, Luchsinger *et al* showed that use of such antibiotics in the general population failed to confer any benefit in terms of presentation of subsequent MI.[32]. Supporting these findings, the ACADEMIC study (Azithromycin in Coronary Artery Disease Elimination of Myocardial Infection with *Chlamydia* study) showed that over a 3 month treatment period, azithromycin failed to prevent adverse cardiovascular events at 6 months and at 2 years[33], despite reducing certain markers of inflammation. The ISAR-3 study randomised patients undergoing coronary stenting to receive roxithromycin or placebo[34]. Although the angiographic restenosis rate and mortality rates were no different between the active and placebo groups the investigators did identify that those patients with highest levels of antibodies to *C pneumoniae* and given the antibiotic had a significant reduction in the rate of restenosis. Clearly the pathology of restenosis differs to that of 'native' atherosclerosis and may not necessarily be an aetiological factor in the former scenario. In another clinical context the expansion rate of abdominal aortic aneurysms was reduced by 43% in a roxithromycin-treated group of patients compared to controls[35].

The anti-*chlamydial* agents, particularly the macrolides used in these early antibiotic intervention studies could be acting through non-antimicrobial effects (e.g. anti-inflammatory actions) thereby halting the progression of atherogenesis /atherothrombosis[36]. Interestingly, other broad-spectrum antibiotics with anti-*chlamydial* activities such as tetracyclines inhibit macrophage matrix metalloproteinases and hence may hypothetically stabilise the atherosclerotic plaque[37]. Several large-scale trials of anti-*chlamydial* antibiotic therapy in various subsets of patients with CHD are currently underway with some 25,000 patients recruited and randomised to receive antibiotic or placebo and under follow up for adverse cardiovascular events[38]. The largest randomised trial (n>7500 subjects), the WIZARD Study[39] (which includes patients recruited from India) has shown a 7% non-significant reduction in major adverse CHD events in post myocardial infarction patients given 3 months of azithromycin therapy – although there seemed to be an early benefit, particularly in diabetics and smokers. The results of two other large trials, ACES and PROVE-IT, will be known in mid-2004.

Infection and atherosclerosis – a current viewpoint

It is plausible that infection, by interacting with the classical risk factors, may predispose certain genetically susceptible individuals to atherosclerosis[40]. Evidence of such a modulatory role for *C pneumoniae* does exist. (*C pneumoniae* prevalence does correlate with hypertension[41], cigarette smoking[42], hyperlipidaemia[43] and male gender). The notion that micro-organisms may cause inflammatory or immune-mediated, non-infectious diseases is not new. *Helicobacter pylori* is now recognised as an aetiological factor in peptic ulceration[44]. Epstein Barr virus has been linked to naso-pharyngeal carcinoma[45]. Mycobacteria have been identified in Crohn's disease[46] and *Tropheryma whippleii* has been linked to Whipple's disease[47]. Although the focus of this review has been on *C pneumoniae* the notion of multiple differing pathogens and 'total pathogen burden' being more contributory to atherosclerosis is also plausible[48].

Despite the current level of interesting evidence there is no doubt that a number of important issues remain unresolved in the 'infectious hypothesis'. The role of antibiotic therapy in CHD also remains controversial[49]. The diagnosis of *C pneumoniae* infection is difficult and there are unclear factors such as re-infection rates, optimal length of antibiotic therapies and dosing regimes in addition to the potential for resistance to anti-microbial therapy emerging.

Infection, inflammation and atherosclerosis – what relevance for South Asians?

To date, from the Indian subcontinent, investigators have correlated an association between markers of chronic *C pneumonaie* infection and CHD[50] (as seen within non-Asian populations). Furthermore CRP appears to be a stronger pathogenetic factor in South Asians than in white Europeans[6]. Such findings tend to propose that both inflammation and infection may have a role in the aetiology and/or progression of CHD in South Asian populations too.

Preliminary work from the UK has shown a close association between both previous exposure to *C pneumonaie* and CRP with angina, as defined by the Rose questionnaire[15] (although no relationship identified between *C. pneumoniae* infection and CRP[51]). Compared with Europeans, subjects of South Asian descent had a greater level of serum gammaglobulin (IgG), a non-specific marker of immune activation - a disparity that remained even when controlling for cigarette smoking[52].

Whether South Asian populations have a greater 'total infectious burden' (potentially fuelling inflammatory processes) or whether hitherto undefined genetic factors and/or altered immune responses (independent of infection) are contributory, merits further research. The link between CRP, dysplipidaemia and the metabolic syndrome illustrates how the multifactorial nature of CHD needs to be extended in exploring the relevance of novel and 'non-traditional risk' atherogenic factors for populations, such as South Asians. Intriguing data also demonstrates that statins and fibrates could exert cardio-protective properties by reducing markers of inflammation and endothelial activation (in addition to the established lipid-lowering effects) - introducing new potential avenues of intervention in those at highest cardiovascular risk and intervention at an early pre-clinical stage.

Conclusion

We need to remind ourselves of the increasing burden of CHD globally. The discovery of 'new' risk factors and novel treatments should not be dismissed without thorough scrutiny. CHD remains the commonest cause of death in the developed world and is projected to continue the trend worldwide. In fact by the year 2020 it is projected that in all regions of the world (including former socialist economies, emerging economies, countries within Indian subcontinent and the Middle East) cardiovascular diseases will become the leading cause of death[1]. Most of these countries will not be able to have access to or fully afford sophisticated and expensive coronary interventions and surgery which the developed world is privileged to. The 'infectious hypothesis' may hence be more relevant in these regions if proven to be true.

Clearly the natural history of *C pneumoniae* infection needs further elucidation as do improvements in diagnosis of and monitoring of infection – but this may have to follow on or be explored in parallel to clinical trials. Results from large-scale trials (and perhaps future trial meta-analyses) may help to clarify the nature of the link between *C pneumoniae* infection and CHD. Perhaps a sub-group of patients might be defined to gain the most benefit from chronic antibiotic therapy – rather than widespread usage amongst all subjects with CHD.

Although a mere coincidental association between *C pneumoniae* infection and CHD is still a possibility the increasing and diverse lines of evidence and CHD are increasing. Definitive proof may only come if subsequent vaccination trials are ever felt to be feasible and can be conducted. We eagerly await the results of the next wave of antibiotic studies. These may go some way to clarify the nature of the link between infection and CHD. Moreover they may help to clarify whether antibiotics have any role, if at all, in the secondary prevention of the 'epidemic' of CHD. We should remain focussed on targeting and treating the established risk factors for CHD using the therapeutic strategies of proven and evidence-based value. No doubt, exciting research lies ahead to confirm or refute the 'infectious' basis to atherosclerosis.

References

1.   Murray CJL, Lopez AD. Mortality by cause for eight regions of the world: global burden of disease study. Lancet 1997;349:1269-76.

2.   Braunwald E. Shattuck lecture- cardiovascular medicine at the turn of the millennium: triumphs, concerns, and opportunities. N Engl J Med 1997;337:1360-69.

3.   Danesh J, Collins R, Peto R. Chronic infections and coronary heart disease: is there a link? Lancet 1997;350:430-36.

4.   Gupta S. Chronic infection in the aetiology of atherosclerosis- focus on Chlamydia pneumoniae. [The John French Memorial Lecture] Atherosclerosis 1999;143:1-6.

5.   Ross R. Atherosclerosis- An inflammatory disease. N Engl J Med 1999;340:115-26.

6.   Chambers J, Eda S, Bassett P et al. C-reactive, insulin resistance, central obesity and coronary heart disease risk in Indian Asians from the United Kingdom compared with European Whites. Circulation 2001; 104: 145-50.

7.   Cook PJ, Honeybourne D. Chlamydia pneumoniae. J Antimicrob Chemother 1994;34:859-73.

8.   Saikku P. The epidemiology and significance of Chlamydia pneumoniae. J Infect 1992;1:27-34.

9.   Saikku P, Mattila K, Nieminen MS et al. Serological evidence of an association of a novel Chlamydia, TWAR, with chronic coronary heart disease and acute myocardial infarction. Lancet 1988;2:983-86.

10.   Gupta S, Camm AJ. Chronic infection, Chlamydia and coronary heart disease. Kluwer Academic Publishers, Dordrecht, 1999. ISBN 0-7923-5797-3.

11.   Wald NJ, Law MR, Morris JK et al. Chlamydia pneumoniae infection and mortality from ischaemic heart disease: large prospective study. BMJ 2000;321:204-7

12.   Danesh J, Whincup P, Walker M et al. Chlamydia pneumoniae IgG titres and coronary heart disease: prospective study and meta-analysis. BMJ 2000;321:208-13.

13.   Shor A, Kuo CC, Patton D. Detection of Chlamydia pneumoniae in coronary arterial fatty streaks and atheromatous plaques. S Afr Med J 1992;82:158-61.

14.   Taylor-Robinson D, Thomas BJ. Chlamydia pneumoniae in arteries: the facts, their interpretation, and future studies. J Clin Pathol 1998;51:793-7.

15. Jackson LA, Campbell LA, Schmidt RA et al. Specificity of detection of Chlamydia pneumoniae in cardiovascular atheroma- evaluation of the innocent bystander hypothesis Am J Pathol 1997;150:1785-90.

16. Kuo CC, Shor A, Campbell LA et al. Demonstration of Chlamydia pneumoniae in atherosclerotic lesions of coronary arteries. J Infect Dis 1993;167:841-9.

17. Ramirez JA. For the Chlamydia pneumoniae / Atherosclerosis Study Group, Isolation of Chlamydia pneumoniae from the coronary artery of a patient with coronary atherosclerosis. Ann Intern Med 1996;125:979-82.

18. Maass M, Bartels C, Engel PM et al. Endovascular presence of viable Chlamydia pneumoniae is a common phenomenon in coronary artery disease. J Am Coll Cardiol 1998;31:827-32.

19. Fabricant CG, Fabricant J, Litrenta MM et al. Virus-induced atherosclerosis. J Exp Med 1978;148:335-340.

20. Fong IW, Chiu B, Viira E et al. Rabbit models for Chlamydia pneumoniae infection. J Clin Microbiol 1997;35:48-52.

21. Muhlestein JB, Anderson JL, Hammond EH et al. Infection with Chlamydia pneumoniae accelerates the development of atherosclerosis and treatment with azithromycin prevents it in a rabbit model. Circulation 1998;97:633-6.

22. Hu H, Pierce GN, Zhong G. The atherogenic effects of chlamydia are dependent on serum cholesterol and specific to Chlamydia pneumoniae. J Clin Invest 1999;103:747-53.

23. Kaukoranta-Tolvanen SS, Teppo AM, Laitinen K et al. Growth of Chlamydia pneumoniae in cultured human peripheral blood mononuclear cells and induction of a cytokine response. Microb Pathog 1996;21:215-21.

24. Kaukoranta-Tolvanen SS, Laitinen K, Saikku P et al. Chlamydia pneumoniae multiplies in human endothelial cells in vitro. Microb Pathog 1994;16:313-9.

25. Gupta S, Camm AJ. Chlamydia pneumoniae and coronary heart disease: coincidence, association or causation? BMJ 1997;314:1778-9.

26. Kol A, Sukhova GK, Lichtman A.H, Libby P. Chlamydia heat shock protein 60 localises in human atheroma and regulates macrophage tumour necrosis factor-α and matrix metalloproteinase expression. Circulation 1998;98:300-7.

27. Gupta S. Chlamydia pneumoniae, monocyte activation and azithromycin in coronary heart disease. Am Heart J 1999;138 Part2 Suppl: S539-41.

28. Gupta S, Leatham EW, Carrington D et al. Elevated Chlamydia pneumoniae antibodies, cardiovascular events and azithromycin in male survivors of myocardial infarction. Circulation 1997;96:404-17.

29. Gurfinkel E, Bozovich G, Daroca A et al. Randomised trial of roxithromycin in non-Q-wave coronary syndromes: ROXIS pilot study. Lancet 1997;350:404-17.

30. Meier CR, Derby LE, Jick SS et al. Antibiotics and risk of subsequent first-time acute myocardial infarction. JAMA 1999;281:427-31.

31. Pilote L, Green L, Joseph L et al. Antibiotics against Chlamydia pneumoniae and prognosis after acute myocardial infarction. Am Heart J 2002;143: 294-300.

32. Luchsinger JA, Pablos-Mendez A, Knirsch C et al. Relation of antibiotic use to risk of myocardial infarction in the general population. Am J Cardiol 2002; 89: 18-20.

33. Muhlestein JB, Anderson JL, Carlquist JF et al. Randomised secondary prevention trial of azithromycin in patients with coronary artery disease: primary clinical results of the ACADEMIC Study. Circulation 2000;102:1755-60.

34. Neumann F, Kastrati A, Miethke T et al. Treatment of Chlamydia pneumoniae infection with roxithromycin and effect on neointima proliferation after coronary stent placement (ISAR-3): a randomised, double-blind, placebo-controlled trial. Lancet 2001;357:2085-9.

35. Vammen S, Lindholt JS, Ostergaard L et al. Randomised double-blind controlled trial of roxithromycin for prevention of abdominal aortic aneurysm expansion. British Journal of Surgery 2001;88:1066-72.

36. Martin D, Bursill J, Qui MR et al. Alternative hypothesis for efficacy of macrolides in acute coronary syndromes. Lancet 1998;351:1858-9.

37. Franklin IJ, Harley SL, Greenhalgh RM, Powell JT. Uptake of tetracycline by aortic aneurysm wall and its effect on inflammation and proteolysis. Br J Surg 1999;86:771-5.

38. Gupta S, Kaski JC. Infections and coronary heart disease: potential for new therapies? Volume II, J Betteridge, eds. Lipids: current perspectives, Martin Dunitz Ltd pubs, May 2000, pp. 107-120.

39. O'Connor C, Dunne M, Pfeffer M et al. Azithromycin for the secondary prevention of coronary heart disease events (WIZARD study): a randomised controlled trial. JAMA 2003;190:1459-66.

40.   Dahlen GH, Boman J, Birgander LS, Lindholm B. Lipoprotein(a), IgG, IgA and IgM antibodies to Chlamydia pneumoniae and HLA class II genotype in early coronary artery disease. Atherosclerosis 1995;114:165-74.

41.   Cook PJ, Lip GY, Davies P et al. Chlamydia pneumoniae antibodies in severe essential hypertension. Hypertension 1998;31:589-94.

42.   Hahn DL, Golubjatnikov R. Smoking is a potential confounder of the Chlamydia pneumoniae-coronary artery disease association. Arterioscler Thromb Vasc Biol1992;12:255-60.

43.   Laurila A, Bloigu A, Nayha S et al. Chronic Chlamydia pneumoniae infection is associated with a serum lipid profile known to be a risk factor for atherosclerosis. Arterioscler Thromb Vasc Biol 1997;17:2910-3.

44.   Marshall BJ. Helicobacter pylori in peptic ulcer: Have Koch's postulates been fulfilled? Ann Med 1995;27:565-8.

45.   Niedobitek G. Epstein-Barr virus infection in the pathogenesis of nasopharyngeal carcinoma. Molecular Pathology 2000;53:248-54.

46.   Sanderson JD, Moss MT, Tizard ML, Hermon-Taylor J. Mycobacterium paratuberculosis DNA in Crohn's disease tissues. Gut 1992;33:890-6.

47.   Ratnaike RN. Whipple's disease. Postgrad Med J 2000;76:760-6.

48.   Rupprecht H, Blankenberg S, Bickel C et al. Impact of viral and bacterial infectious burden on long-term prognosis in patients with coronary artery disease. Circulation 2001;104:25-31.

49.   Anand V, Gupta S. Antibiotic therapy in coronary heart disease - where do we currently stand? Cardiovascular Drugs and Therapy 2001;15:209-10.

50.   Bahl V, Sengupta P, Sathpathy G et al. Chlamydia pneumoniae infection and non-specifc aortoartereritis: search for a link with a nonatherosclerotic inflammatory arterial disease. Indian Heart J 2002; 54: 46-9.

51.   Fischbacher C, Bhopal R, Todd A et al. Chlamydia pneumoniae IgG titres and coronary heart disease: prospective study and meta-analysis. Consider ethnic variations. BMJ 2000 (rapid response, Letter)

52.   Fischbacher C, Bhopal R , Blackwell C et al. IgG is higher in south Asians than Europeans: does infection contribute to ethnic variation in cardiovascular disease? Arterioscler Thromb Vasc Biol 2003; 23: 703-4

8

Nutrition and coronary heart disease in South Asians

T A B Sanders

Overview

The diets of the UK South Asian population are diverse, ranging from strict vegetarian to meat and fish containing diets. Despite this dietary diversity, central obesity and insulin resistance is more prevalent in all groups when compared to the white population. Total dietary fat intakes are similar to those in the white population but the intake of linoleic acid tends to be higher because of the widespread use of oils. Vegetarian groups are likely to have low intakes of vitamin B_{12} which can result in elevated plasma homocysteine concentrations. Low dietary intakes of vitamin D coupled with low sunlight exposure may also be related to risk of CHD. Dietary advice to decrease the intake of saturated fatty acids is prudent but advice to decrease total fat intake and increase carbohydrate intake may exacerbate insulin resistance. Emerging evidence suggests that advice to consume a diet rich in carbohydrates with a low glycaemic index may have favourable effects on insulin resistance. There is some evidence that an increased intake of fruit and vegetables, nuts and oils rich in linolenic acid may decrease risk of CHD. However, avoiding obesity and taking moderate daily physical activity should probably remain the cornerstone of dietary advice for the prevention of CHD in the South Asian community.

Introduction

As already discussed in earlier chapters, The UK population of approximately 1.6 million people of South Asian ethnic origin has a higher CHD mortality risk compared to the white population. Young South Asian males account for a substantial proportion of this excess. CHD mortality is particularly high in postmenopausal South Asian women (see Chapter 1). The dietary habits of the South Asian population are relatively diverse and are influenced by religious belief as well as area of origin in the Indian sub-continent. According to the 2001 census 1.1% of the total population in England stated they were of Hindu faith, a faith which advocates a vegetarian diet. Muslims do not eat pork and Sikhs may only eat meat that has been ritually slaughtered. Generally South Asian diets are cereal based but the staple food consumed depends on the area from which South Asians originate. Wheat is predominately grown in the North part of the sub-continent, therefore Punjabis and Sikhs consume more wheat. Chicken and lamb/goat are the preferred meats in these groups. Bangladeshis are known to prefer rice as it is the main crop cultivated in the Ganges delta. Fish is also more popular with Bangladeshis than other South Asian groups. Gujaratis consume rice, wheat and also millet.

As discussed earlier, conventional risk factors alone do not explain the excess CHD mortality in South Asians (see Chapter 2). It is thought that glucose intolerance and hyperinsulinaemia account for much of the excess prevalence of CHD, consistent with the hypothesis that metabolic disturbances associated with insulin resistance underlie the high risk in South Asians[1].

Dietary Patterns

The National Food Survey[2] which records household food purchases suggests lower total fat intake, higher total polyunsaturated fatty acid intake and a higher polyunsaturated: saturated fatty acid intake ratio in South Asians than in whites. However, this survey fails to take into account the diverse nature of different South Asian diets. Lack of detailed information on ethnicity has meant that the larger population surveys have been unable to successfully identify the diets of South Asian households. Detailed measurements of dietary intake and an evaluation of dietary intake have been made using 7-day weighed food intakes[3,4]. The proportion of energy derived from fat in South Asian diet is comparable or slightly lower than that in the general population[5]. Vegetable oils such as corn oil are predominantly used for cooking and this explains the relatively higher intake of the polyunsaturated fatty acid, linoleic acid. Studies have generally found that dietary intakes are closer to the recommended dietary intakes with regard to saturated fatty acids than those of the general population particularly in Gujaratis (Table 8.1). Dietary intakes of cholesterol are lower and the intake of polyunsaturated fatty acids (PUFA), particularly linoleic acid is much higher in the Gujarati population, who show high levels of vegetarianism compared with the general population. However, intakes of saturated fatty acids are generally more similar to the general population in muslims because of their intake of fatty meats such as lamb and beef. This is notable in the Bangladeshi community in London where the intake of total and saturated fatty acids is relatively high[5] and is mainly attributable to their preference for lamb and beef, which are fatty meats high in saturated fatty acids.

It is important to recognise that dietary habits are changing and the data derived from the migrant generation may not necessarily apply to offspring born in the UK who have food habits which have become more representative of general population UK food habits[5,6]. A major limitation to estimating dietary intake in the South Asian community has been the lack of reliable food composition data. However, a jointly funded project by the Agha Khan Foundation and the Department of Health has now published tables of food composition that will help estimate dietary intake in Asian diets[7].

Table 8.1: Dietary intakes measured in South Asian men and women (predominantly of Gujarati origin) as determined by 7-day weighed food intake records in North London (Data from Miller et al[3] and Reddy & Sanders[4])

	Males		Females	
	South Asian	White	South Asian	White
Energy intake MJ/d	9.3	11.2	6.1	7.5
Protein (% energy)	12.6	14.3	11.7	15.8
Fat (% energy)	38.4	38.2	37.3	40.3
P/S ratio	0.52	0.26	0.66	0.41
Carbohydrate (% energy)	46.5	43.8	54	43
Fibre (g/day)	27.8	23.1	16.6	16.2

A substantial proportion of the South Asian population who are Hindus follows a vegetarian diet and consequently has low intakes of vitamin B_{12}. Combined folate and vitamin B_{12} deficiency resulting in megaloblastic anaemic were more common in the South Asian vegetarian population and subsequent studies have shown that elevated homocysteine (Hcy) concentrations are more strongly associated with low serum vitamin B_{12} concentrations than with serum folate[8]. Although, a systematic review suggests that elevated plasma Hcy is associated with increased risk of CHD[9], the difference in Hcy levels between South Asians and whites is not sufficient to explain the difference in CHD risk. Furthermore, UK white vegetarians have been found to have elevated plasma Hcy concentrations[10] due to vitamin B_{12} deficiency but to have a lower risk of CHD compared with the omnivores[11].

The type of fatty acids consumed in South Asian diets is quite variable. Vegetarian diets tend to contain a high proportion of linoleic acid and are usually devoid of long-chain n-3 fatty acids. This results in lower levels of n-3 fatty acids in their blood lipids[3,4]. Several large cohort studies have found a relationship between lower intakes of long-chain n-3 fatty acids and increased risk of fatal cardiovascular disease and randomised controlled trials have found that an increased intake of n-3 fatty acids resulted in a significant reduction in fatal CHD[12]. A study of an Indo-Mediterranean diet conducted in India suggested that an increased intake of fruit and vegetables, nuts and linolenic acid reported decreased incidence of fatal CHD[13].

Research conducted in the Bangladeshi community in East London has revealed a strikingly different dietary pattern compared with the predominantly vegetarian Gujarati population. In this group intakes of saturated fatty acids tend to be higher and the intake of fish is popular[14]. Boucher[15] has suggested that the low intake of vitamin D in the Asian population may be related to increased risk of CHD. In the UK there was an epidemic of "Asian rickets" in the early 1970's. The reasons for the decline in rickets are complex but in part it may be due to an increased calcium intake and a decline in the consumption of phytic acid rich foods. Serum vitamin D concentrations, however, still remain low in many Asians[16]. Boucher's group[15] has recently shown that vitamin D supplementation decreases the activity of matrix metalloproteinase-9 (MMP-9), which could be of significance with regard to risk of CHD. MMP-9 is believed to be involved in increasing susceptibility to plaque rupture (as discussed by Shah and Kearney in chapter 4).

Diet and insulin resistance

Measurements of fat patterning have been able to discriminate differences between children of South Asian origin compared with whites and it is possible to detect early signs of insulin resistance in South Asian children. Pioneering studies carried out by Miller[17] in the Caribbean showed that men of South Asian origin had lower concentrations of HDL cholesterol and higher plasma insulin concentrations compared with other ethnic groups and that this was associated with increased risk of CHD. These findings have been replicated in other communities originating from the subcontinent of Asia, for example in Singapore and South Africa. General dietary advice that emphasises a substantial reduction in total fat intake and a large increase in carbohydrate intake may be less appropriate for the Asian population. Indeed such dietary interventions have been found to result in an increase in plasma triglyceride concentration and a reduction of in HDL cholesterol concentration which is consistent with increased insulin resistance[18].

Life-style interventions to reduce risk of CHD in South Asians

The key issue with regard to the prevention of CHD in the South Asian community is probably to modify lifestyle factors that decrease the consequences associated with insulin resistance. There is convincing evidence[19] that moderate physical activity and a decrease in body weight improve insulin sensitivity and features of insulin resistance. However the role of dietary fat composition is less certain. Diets high in saturated fatty acids probably exacerbate insulin resistance[20] and given their plasma cholesterol raising effect, there is consensus on the need to decrease population intakes of saturated fatty acids. However, an issue of dietary carbohydrate quality and specifically, the glycaemic index of carbohydrate[21] may be of particular importance. Indeed, there is some evidence of an improvement in insulin sensitivity in South Asian subjects advised to follow a diet with a low glycaemic index[22]. The glycaemic index can be lowered by replacing starchy foods such as ordinary rice and chappatis with versions that have a lower glycaemic index and by decreasing the intake of sugary foods. Interestingly the glycaemic index of a food such as rice is dependent on its source and how it is processed. Wholegrain cereals usually have a lower glycaemic index than refined cereals (except for bread). Basmati rice and parboiled rice have a substantially lower glycaemic index compared with ordinary boiled rice. The pattern in which food is consumed also has an impact on insulin sensitivity – with smaller doses spread throughout the day having a more favourable effect than the consumption of a large amount in a single meal. Consequently, in order to modify the overall glycaemic index of a diet requires altering both the pattern of carbohydrate intake as well as the type of carbohydrate consumed.

Conclusion

The Department of Health COMA panel[23] made several recommendations for the prevention of CHD in the UK. However, these did not specifically cover the needs of the South Asian population, for whom translation of this advice needs to be refined. There is also a need to develop a sounder scientific basis for dietary advice for the prevention of CHD in the South Asian population. The current knowledge suggests that it is prudent to restrict the intakes of saturated fatty acids and to encourage an increased intake of fruit and vegetables and oils rich in linolenic acid. There is promising research that suggests that decreasing the glycaemic index of the diet may be of value in preventing/managing insulin resistance but further research in this area is needed. These aspects of diet coupled with regular physical activity, avoidance of obesity and decreasing the intake of saturated fatty acids are currently the most effective diet related life-style interventions with regard to decreasing risk of cardiovascular disease[24].

References

1.   McKeigue PM, Shah B, Marmot MG. Relation of central obesity and insulin resistance with high diabetes prevalence and cardiovascular risk in South Asians. Lancet 1991; 337: 382-386.

2.   National Food Survey. http:// statistics. defra. gov.uk /esg /publications /nfs /default.asp Accessed 10/06/03

3.   Miller GJ, Kotecha S, Wilkinson WH, Wilkes H, Stirling Y, Sanders TA, Broadhurst A, Allison J, Meade TW. Dietary and other characteristics relevant for coronary heart disease in men of Indian, West Indian and European descent in London. Atherosclerosis 1988;70:63-72.

4.   Reddy S, Sanders TA. Lipoprotein risk factors in vegetarian women of Indian descent are unrelated to dietary intake. Atherosclerosis 1992;95:223-9.

5.   Landman J, Cruickshank K. A review of the ethnicity, health and nutrition-related diseases in relation to migration in the United Kingdom. Public Health Nutrition 2001;4:647-657.

6.   Thomas J. Nutrition intervention in ethnic minority groups. Proc.Nutr.Soc. 2002;61:559-67.

7.   Judd PA, Kassam-Khamis T, Thomas JE. The composition and nutrient content of foods commonly consumed by South Asians in the UK. Tha Agha Khan Board for the UK. London, 2000.

8.   Chambers JC, Kooner JS. Homocysteine: a novel risk factor for coronary heart disease in UK Indian Asians. Heart 2001;86:121-2.

9.   Wald DS, Law M, Morris JK. Homocysteine and cardiovascular disease: evidence on causality from a meta-analysis. BMJ 2002;325:1202.

10.   Lloyd-Wright Z, Hvas A, Møller A, Sanders TA, Nexo E. Holotranscobalamin – an indicator of dietary vitamin B12 deficiency. Clini Chem (in press)

11.   Key TJ, Fraser GE, Thorogood M, Appleby PN, Beral V, Reeves G et al. Mortality in vegetarians and nonvegetarians: detailed findings from a collaborative analysis of 5 prospective studies. Am.J.Clin.Nutr. 1999;70(Suppl):516S-24S.

12.   Hu FB, Willett WC: Optimal diets for prevention of coronary heart disease. *JAMA* 2002, 288: 2569-2578.

13.   Singh RB, Dubnov G, Niaz MA, Ghosh S, Singh R, Rastogi SS, Manor O, Pella D, Berry EM. Effect of an Indo-Mediterranean diet on progression of coronary artery disease in high risk patients (Indo-Mediterranean Diet Heart Study): a randomised single-blind trial. Lancet 2002;360:1455-61.

14.   McKeigue PM, Marmot MG, Syndercombe Court YD, Cottier DE, Rahman S, Riemersma RA. Diabetes, hyperinsulinaemia, and coronary risk factors in Bangladeshis in east London. Br.Heart J. 1988;60:390-6.

15.   Timms PM, Mannan N, Hitman GA, Noonan K, Mills PG, Syndercombe-Court, Aganna E, Price CP, Boucher BJ. Circulating MMP9, vitamin D and variation in the

TIMP-1 response with VDR genotype: mechanisms for inflammatory damage in chronic disorders? QJM. 2002;95:787-96.

16. Serhan E, Holland MR. Relationship of hypovitaminosis D and secondary hyperparathyroidism with bone mineral density among UK resident Indo-Asians. Ann Rheum Dis. 2002 ;61:456-8.

17. Miller GJ, Beckles GL, Alexis SD, Byam NT, Price SG. Serum lipoproteins and susceptibility of men of Indian descent to coronary heart disease. The St James Survey, Trinidad. Lancet 1982;2:200-3.

18. Knopp RH, Retzlaff B, Walden C, Fish B, Buck B, McCann B. One-year effects of increasingly fat-restricted, carbohydrate-enriched diets on lipoprotein levels in free-living subjects. Proc.Soc.Exp.Biol.Med. 2000;225:191-9.

19. Costacou T, Mayer-Davis EJ. Nutrition and Prevention of Type 2 Diabetes. Annu.Rev.Nutr. 2003.

20. Vessby B, Unsitupa M, Hermansen K et al. Substituting dietary saturated for monounsaturated fat impairs insulin sensitivity in healthy men and women: The KANWU Study. Diabetologia 2001;44:312-9.

21. Ludwig DS: The glycemic index: physiological mechanisms relating to obesity, diabetes, and cardiovascular disease. JAMA 2002, 287:2414-2423.

22. Frost G, Leeds A, Trew G, Margara R, Dornhorst A. Insulin sensitivity in women at risk of coronary heart disease and the effect of a low glycemic diet. Metabolism 1998;47:1245-51.

23. Department of Health. Cardiovascular Review Group. Committee on Medical Aspects of Food Policy. Nutritional aspects of cardiovascular disease. Dept of Health Report on Health and Social Services, 46. London, HMSO, 1994.

24. Executive Summary of The Third Report of The National Cholesterol Education Program (NCEP) Expert Panel on Detection, Evaluation, And Treatment of High Blood Cholesterol In Adults (Adult Treatment Panel III). JAMA 2001, 285:2486-2497

9

Hypertension and coronary heart disease in South Asians

C Agyemang and R S Bhopal

Introduction

Coronary heart disease and stroke are dominant causes of death in South Asian populations in the UK and the rates are even higher than in the white population[1]. As a major cardiovascular risk factor, hypertension needs to be carefully managed in South Asian populations. There is a perception that in South Asians blood pressures are comparatively high. Studies in the UK on comparisons between South Asian and white populations in blood pressure and prevalence of hypertension have, however, given inconsistent conclusions. This chapter discusses blood pressure and prevalence of hypertension data on samples of South Asian populations in the community in comparison with a white or general population in the UK.

Blood pressure levels

The common perception that blood pressure in South Asians is comparatively high is unreliable – the picture is more complex than this. Overall, blood pressures are similar but there is stark heterogeneity in South Asian adults with slightly higher blood pressures in Indians, slightly lower blood pressures in Pakistanis and much lower blood pressures in Bangladeshis. The available data on blood pressure and prevalence of hypertension in the UK show that most studies reported lower mean systolic but higher diastolic blood pressures in South Asians in both males and females compared to whites[2]. For example, of the 13 community based studies (Table 9.1) in the UK analysed[3-15], 8 reported lower mean systolic blood pressure[3,4,8,9,11,12,14,15] and 7 reported higher mean diastolic blood pressure[3,5,7,9,10,12,13] in South Asian males compared to white males. Of the 9 studies on females[6,7,9-14], 6 reported a lower mean systolic blood pressure[4,6,9,11-13] and 5 reported a higher diastolic blood pressure[7,9,10,12,13] in South Asians compared to whites.

Table 9.1. Blood pressure levels (mean) and prevalence (%) by ethnic group (this table draws upon the table in reference 2 with permission from the Journal of Human Hypertension)

FIRST AUTHOR & PUBLICATION DATE	PLACE OF STUDY	ETHNIC GROUPS	MALES			FEMALES		
			SBP	DBP	% PH	SBP	DBP	% PH
Cruickshank (1983)[3]	Birmingham	Whites	134.2*	78.7	22%	Not studied		
		Asian origin	128.7	79.9*	17%			
McKeigue (1988)[4]	London	Non-Asians	129***	81	Not given	123*	78	Not given
		Bangladeshi	119	78		113	78	
Miller (1988)[5]	London	Europeans	138.0	86.1	21%	Not studied		
		Indians	141.5	88.4	40%			
Cruickshank (1991)[6]	London	Whites	129	77	20%	128	75	34%
		Gujarati Indians	137	77	32%	123	66	13%
McKeigue et al (1991)[7]	London	Europeans	121	78	Not given	120	76	Not given
		South Asians	126	82		126	77	
Knight (1992)[8]	Bradford	Non-Asians	137.4**	79.6	23.1%	Not studied		
		Asians	131.4	79.5	26.6%*			
Williams (1993)[9]	Glasgow	Gen. Population	124.5	80.3	14%	115.3	74.0	5%
		South Asians	123.8	86.3**	22%	111.3	74.5	5%
Cappuccio (1998)[10]	London				WHO JNC			WHO JNC
		Whites	127.9	82.1	28% 18%	123.5	77.2	24% 13%
		South Asians	131.0**	85.4***	44% 33%	127.9***	79.8***	36% 26%
Bhopal (1999)[11]	Newcastle upon Tyne	Europeans	129.1***	78.1**	18%	121.2***	68.8	12%
		South Asians	119.2	70.6	10%	117.7	67.9	14%
		Subgroups:						
		Indians	123.9	72.1	14%	122.6	68.4	15%
		Pakistanis	119.0	70.9	9%	115.7	68.0	12%
		Bangladeshis	112.1	67.5	6%	108.8	66.4	5%
Whitty (1999)[12]	London	Whites	123.4**	76.8	OR 1	120.0	75.0	
		South Asians	121.4	77.4	OR 2.3	119.5	75.4	
				males & females mixed				
Primastesta (2000)[13]	England	Whites						
		16-39	132.2**	70.3	4%	122.8**	68.1	2%
		40 and above	141.6	81.5	36%	138.0	75.8	35%
		South Asians						
		16-39	129.5	71.9	3%	118.9	67.2	2%
		40 and above	143.5	84.1***	51%***	137.9	77.1	33%
Karlsen (2001)[14]	England		SRM	SRM	SRR	SRM		SRR
		Gen. population	136.8 1	76.2 1	40.8% 1	132.5 1		32.9% 1
		Indian	134.0 1.0	77.7 1.03	35.7% 1.03	126.2 0.99		23.6% 1.12
		Pakistani	129.7 0.98	72.5 0.99	25.5% 0.89	122.9 1.02		16.1% 1.25
		Bangladeshi	126.5 0.94	72.9 0.99	23.6% 0.74	120.2 0.97		12.3% 0.89
						DBP not given but similar		
Lane (2002)[15]	England	Whites	129.5	80.4	19.4%	Not studied		
		South Asian	127.6	79.5	16.0%			

SBP = Systolic Blood Pressure, DBP = Diastolic Blood Pressure, BP = Blood Pressure, SRM = Standardized ratios of means, SRR = Standardized Risk Ratio, % PH = Prevalence of Hypertension, (WHO) criteria = BP≥160/95 mm Hg or on drug therapy, (JNC) criteria = BP≥140/90 or on drug therapy, *p<0.05, ** p<0.01, *** p<0.001, comparing ethnic groups

Prevalence of hypertension

Whilst more studies have reported higher prevalence rates of hypertension in South Asian males compared to white males, the prevalence rates in South Asian and white females have shown inconclusive results. For example, of the 11 studies on the prevalence of hypertension using various cut-off points[3,5,6,8-15], 5 reported higher[5,6,8,9,10] and 3 studies reported lower[3,11,15] prevalence rates in South Asian males compared to white males. In Primatesta et al, the prevalence rate was lower in the 16-39 year group but higher in the 40 and above year group compared to whites[13]. In Karlsen et al's study, the observed prevalence of hypertension was lower in South Asian groups than in whites. However, after adjusting for the effects of age and presenting data in the form of relative risk ratios (comparing each sub-group to the overall general population), the age standardised risk ratios were lower in Bangladeshi and Pakistani males but higher in Indian males than in white males[14]. Of 6 studies reported on females[6,9-11,13,14], 2 showed higher prevalence rates[10,11], 1 showed the same rates[9] and 2 showed lower rates[6,13] in South Asians compared with whites. Bhopal et al[11] found the prevalence in Bangladeshi females to be much lower than in Europeans. In Karlsen et al's study, the observed prevalence rates were lower in South Asian groups. However, after the effect of age has been controlled for, the age standardised risk ratios were higher in Pakistani and Indian females but lower in Bangladeshi females compared to white females[14]. Whitty et al's study result was based on males and females combined and reported higher rates in South Asians than in whites[12].

Both mean blood pressure and the prevalence of hypertension data show important differences between South Asian subgroups[11,14] yet most studies combined them as one homogenous group. Data also show regional variation between the London area and the rest of the UK. While lower blood pressure in Bangladeshis was associated with a lower BMI, differences in obesity clearly did not account for much of the ethnic variation[2]. In three studies[16-18] based on clinically selected patients study, hence excluded by Agyemang and Bhopal's systematic review[2], blood pressure levels were lower in South Asian populations than in the white population.

The problems of comparison in UK studies

Results of the UK studies are not clear-cut. Inconsistent results could be explained by differential representation in sample populations by Indians, Pakistanis and Bangladeshis and variations in the methodology of different studies. These factors make inter-study comparisons unreliable and hence intra-study variations between ethnic subgroups are more important. The importance of heterogeneity among South Asian groups has long been emphasised but generally neglected[19]. Variations in South Asian subgroups are especially important in the context of cardiovascular diseases, where risk factor profiles and disease outcomes differ too[11,20]. Heterogeneity among the UK ethnic groups study populations may be a general explanation for inconsistent results from prevalence of hypertension studies.

Huge variations in methods of measurement of blood pressure limit the capacity to synthesise UK data. For example, in some studies, participants' blood pressures were measured with a Hawksley random zero sphygmomanometer[3-7,9]. In other studies[13,14] a Dinamap 8100 monitor was used which tends to provide higher systolic and lower diastolic blood pressure levels than mercury sphygmomanometer readings[21,22]. Participants' blood pressures were measured in different locations and the cut-off point used for diagnosis of hypertension varied too. The estimated effect of whitecoat hypertension ranges from 12 to 53 % depending upon the population studied and definition used[23,24]. It is difficult to account for the effect of whitecoat hypertension in each study. It is also not clear whether the effect of whitecoat hypertension differs in different ethnic groups[25]. The UK studies span approximately 20 years, which potentially affects the comparability and interpretability of results. Middle-aged South Asians at the end of the 20th century were also likely to be different from their counterparts in the early 1980's, with respect to immigration, behaviour and socio-economic status. Differences in BMI, age and sex further complicate the findings of the UK studies.

Some studies[5,6,7] used country of birth as an indicator of ethnicity. This implies that many Indians, Pakistanis and Bangladeshis who were born in the UK were excluded.

Heterogeneity by ethnic subgroup and region

The Newcastle Health Project study and the Health Survey for England '99 are the two studies that paid particular attention to the heterogeneity of the South Asian populations in the UK[11,14]. The Newcastle study found major differences among South Asian subgroups. Bangladeshi males and females had lower mean systolic and diastolic blood pressures than Indian and Pakistani males. Prevalence of hypertension was less common in Bangladeshis in both males and females than in Indian and Pakistani groups[11]. In the recent Health Survey for England '99 similar findings emerged. Bangladeshi males and females had lower age-standardised mean systolic and diastolic blood pressure and a lower prevalence of hypertension than their Indian and Pakistani counterparts[14]. These two studies emphasise the importance of studying South Asian subgroups separately rather than combining them as one homogeneous group, which may make other studies misleading. For example, McKeigue *et al's*[7] study classified South Asian subgroups on the basis of language and religion. This study found significantly higher systolic blood pressure in Sikh (128 mm Hg n=731) and Punjabi Hindus (128 mm Hg n=159) than in Muslims (120 mm Hg n=211) and Gujarati Hindus (122 mm Hg n=127). Despite these differences they were combined as one group.

The UK data also show a regional variation between the London area (comparatively high blood pressure in South Asian males) and the rest of the UK (comparatively lower or similar blood pressure). Most studies in London show higher mean systolic[5-7,10] and diastolic[5,7,10,12] blood pressures in South Asian males than in white males. By contrast, all studies[3,8,9,11,15] in cities outside London show lower mean systolic blood pressure in South Asian males compared to white males. Prevalence data also show similar patterns in South Asian males. Higher blood pressure levels reported in the London area as opposed to other cities outside London may reflect different environmental risk factors experienced by ethnic groups living in different parts of the UK or perhaps more likely, a different population mix. It is possible that London studies which reported higher blood pressure levels in South Asians might have consisted mainly of Indians. For example, Cruickshank *et al's*[6] and McKeigue *et al's*[7] studies reported higher blood pressure levels in South Asian groups. McKeigue *et al's* study drew a large part of the South Asian sample from 16 general-practices in the London borough of Ealing. This borough is composed of 16.1% of Indians (many of them Sikh Punjabis)[26]. Also, in Cruickshank *et al's* [6] study, the South Asian subjects were mainly Gujarati Indians. In contrast, in McKeigue *et al's* [7] study in the London borough of Tower Hamlets with a predominantly Bangladeshi population[26] blood pressure levels were lower compared to whites.

The studies that have a representative sample of the adult population show lower or similar blood pressure levels in South Asian males compared to white males[3,8,11,13,14]. By contrast, most studies on older adults show higher blood pressures[5,6,7,10,13] and higher prevalence rates[5,6,10,13] in South Asian males than in whites. Primatesta *et al's* study had a representative sample of both younger and older adult populations[12]. The older South Asian males group had a higher blood pressure and a higher prevalence rate but the younger South Asian males group had a lower mean systolic blood pressure and lower prevalence rate than white males[12]. It may be that the younger generation of South Asian groups have different blood pressure patterns than the previous generation. Our preliminary observations on South Asian children indicate that the heterogeneity has diminished with Bangladeshi children not enjoying the comparatively low blood pressure their parents have[27].

Blood pressure, prevalence of hypertension and pulse pressure

A higher prevalence of hypertension was not always associated with higher blood pressure in that population. For example, Miller *et al's* study reported a marked excess of hypertension in Indian males but average blood pressure levels were similar in all ethnic groups[5]. Again, in Knight *et al's* study, the prevalence of hypertension was higher in South Asian than non-South Asian males but systolic blood pressure was higher in non-Asians[8]. The possible explanation for this is that either the percentage on antihypertensive treatment differs or the distribution of blood pressure is skewed. In Miller *et al's* study a larger number of Indians were on antihypertensive therapy compared to whites ($p<0.05$)[5].

A lower mean systolic blood pressure but a higher mean diastolic blood pressure reported in South Asians in both males and females implies lower pulse pressure. Evidence on pulse pressure as a marker of cardiovascular risk is well established especially CHD[28,29]. This finding of lower pulse pressure in this review is in direct contrast with the evidence of higher coronary events in South Asian populations particularly in Bangladeshis[20].

Blood pressure and disease outcomes

A meta-analysis of nine major prospective studies has shown an important association between increased blood pressure and stroke and CHD[30]. There are some problems in extrapolating these data to all ethnic groups, as it is unknown whether the physiological optimal level of blood pressure is the same in each group[31]. For example, it remains uncertain whether for a given level of blood pressure South Asian populations will have a higher risk of death than white people. Findings from the St James Study in Trinidad showed that the attributable mortality (the sum of the products of attributable risk and age-adjusted prevalence in each pressure group) after 8 years (in deaths/1000 person years) from a systolic blood pressure between 155 and 179 mm Hg was 12.3 for Indian and 8.2 for European males, and above 180 mm Hg, 22.8 and 15.1 respectively[32]. Bangladeshis have a lower mean systolic and diastolic blood pressure than Indians and Pakistanis[11,14], but a higher mortality from stroke than their Indian and Pakistani counterparts[20]. These differences may be a result of an interaction between risk factors. Among South Asian sub-groups it may be that for a given level of blood pressure the Bangladeshis will have higher risk of death than Indians or Pakistanis. These findings seem to suggest that the reporting of blood pressure and distributions is better than using arbitrary cut-off points.

Conclusion

Blood pressure levels and prevalence of hypertension differ across groups. Some of the inconsistent results in the UK studies could be explained by the variations in methods of measurement of blood pressure and classifications of South Asian groups. Differences in age, sex and BMI also potentially confound findings. A growing proportion of people from India, Pakistan and Bangladesh origin are UK born. There is therefore a strong case for epidemiological research among younger groups to examine blood pressure levels and prevalence of hypertension and how this pattern may be changing. The early observations are a warning[27]. Future research must recognise the various subgroups of South Asians and should be designed in such a way that data can be combined easily, for example by standardising the way in which blood pressure is measured. Given the observations on blood pressure levels and the risks of stroke and CHD, clinicians need to tackle hypertension, and its causes, with the utmost vigour.

Acknowledgements

We thank again the people acknowledged in reference 2. This paper relies heavily upon that paper with permission of the Journal of Human Hypertension.

References

1.   Bhopal R, Sengupta-Wiebe S. Cardiovascular risks and outcomes: ethnic variations in hypertensive patients. Heart 2000; 83: 495-496

2.   Agyemang C, Bhopal R S. Is blood pressure of South Asian adults in the UK higher or lower than that in European white adults? A review of cross-sectional data, Journal of Human Hypertension 2002; 16: 739-751

3.   Cruickshank JK et al. Blood pressure in black, white and Asian factory workers in Birmingham. Postgrad Med J 1983; 59: 622-626

4.   McKeigue PM et al. Diabetes, hyperinsulinaemia, and coronary risk factors in Bangladeshis in East London. Br Heart J 1988; 60: 390-396

5.   Miller GJ et al. Dietary and other characteristics relevant for coronary heart disease in males of Indian, West Indian and European descent in London. Atherosclerosis 1988; 70: 63-72

6.   Cruickshank JK et al. Ethnic differences in fasting plasma C-peptide and insulin in relation to glucose tolerance and blood pressure. Lancet 1991; 338: 842-847

7.   McKeigue PM, Shah B, Marmot MG. Relation of central obesity and insulin resistance with high diabetes prevalence and cardiovascular risk in South Asians. Lancet 1991; 337: 382-386

8.   Knight TM et al. Insulin resistance, diabetes, and risk markers for ischaemic heart disease in Asian males and non-Asian males in Bradford. Br Heart J 1992; 67: 343-350

9.   Williams R, Bhopal R, Hunt K. Health of a Punjabi ethnic minority in Glasgow: a comparison with the general population, J Epidemiol and Community Health 1993; 47: 96-102

10.   Cappuccio FP, Cooj DG, Atkinson RW, Wicks PD. The Wandsworth Heart and Stroke Study. A population-based survey of cardiovascular risk factors in different ethnic groups. Methods and baseline findings. Nutr Metab Cardiovasc Dis 1998; 8: 371-385

11.   Bhopal R et al. Heterogeneity of coronary heart disease risk factors in Indian, Pakistani, Bangladeshi, and European origin populations: cross sectional study. BMJ 1999; 319: 215-220

12.   Whitty CJM et al. Differences in biological risk factors for cardiovascular disease between three ethnic groups in the Whitehall II study. Atherosclerosis 1999; 142: 279-286

13.   Primatesta P, Bost L, Poulter NR. Blood pressure levels and hypertension status among ethnic groups in England. Journal of Human Hypertension 2000; 14: 143-148

14.   Karlsen S, Primatesta P, McMum A. Blood Pressure. Chapter 7 In: Erens B, Primatesta P, Prior G. Health Survey for England – The Health of Minority Ethnic Groups '99 London. The Stationary Office, 2001, pp 175-197

15.   Lane D, Beevers DG, Lip GYH. Ethnic differences in blood pressure and prevalence of hypertension in England, Journal of Human Hypertension 2002; 16: 267-273

16.   Pacy PJ et al. Prevalence of Hypertension in White, Black and Asian Diabetic in a District Hospital Diabetic Clinic. Diabetic Medicine 1984; 2: 125-130

17.   Hughes LO, Cruickshank JK, Wright J, Raftery EB. Disturbances of insulin in British Asians and white males surviving myocardial infarction. BMJ 1989; 299: 537-541

18.   Khattar R.S, Swales JD, Senior R, Lahiri A. Racial variation in cardiovascular morbidity and mortality in essential hypertension, Heart 2000; 83: 267-271

19.   Bhopal RS, Phillimore P, Kohli HS. Inappropriate use of the term "Asians": an obstacle to ethnicity and health research. J Pub Health Med 1991; 13: 244-246

20.   Gill PS, Kai J, Bhopal RS, Wild S. Health Care Needs Assessment: Black and Minority Ethnic Groups. In: Raftery J (ed). Health Care Needs Assessment. The epidemiologically based needs assessment reviews. Third Series. Abingdon: Radcliffe Medical Press Ltd. (in press) http://hcna.radcliffe-online.com/bemgframe.htm

21. Weaver MG, Park MK, Lee KH. Difference in Blood Pressure Levels Obtained by Auscultatory and Oscillometric Methods. Am J Dis Child 1990; 144: 911-914

22. Bolling K. Dinamap 8100 caribration study, OPCS: London, HMSO, 1994

23. Pickering TG et al. How common is white coat hypertension? Journal of the American Medical Association 1988; 259: 225-228

24. Verdecchia P. Variability between current definition of 'normal' ambulatory blood pressure: implications in the assessment of white coat hypertension. Hypertension 1992; 20: 555-562

25. Agyemang C, Bhopal R S. Is the blood pressure of people from African origin adults in the UK higher or lower than that in European origin whites? A review of cross-sectional data, Journal of Human Hypertension 2003; 17: 523-534

26. Owen, D. 91 Census statistical papers 1–9, Warwick: Centre for Research in Ethnic Relations, University of Warwick/CRE, 1992-1995

27. Agyemang C, Bhopal R, Bruijnzeels M. Do variations in blood pressure of ethnic minority children reflect those of the adult populations in the UK? A review of cross-sectional data (in press)

28. Madhavan S et al. Relation of pulse pressure and blood pressure reduction to the incidence of myocardial infarction. Hypertension 1994; 23: 395-401

29. Stanley S et al. Is Pulse Pressure Useful in Predicting Risk for Coronary Heart Disease? The Framingham Heart Study. Circulation 1999; 100: 354-360

30. MacMahon S, Peto R, Cutler J. Blood pressure, stroke, and coronary heart disease, Part 1, prolonged differences in blood pressure: prospective observational studies corrected for the regression dilution biases, Lancet 1990; 335: 765-774

31. McKeigue, P.M., & Sevak, L. Coronary Heart Disease in South Asian Communities. London: Health Education Authority, 1994

32. Miller GJ et al. Adult Male All-Cause, Cardiovascular and Cerebrovascular Mortality in Relation to Ethnic Group, Systolic Blood Pressure and Blood Glucose Concentration in Trinidad, West Indies Inter J Epidemiol 1988; 17: 62-69

10

Smoking and smoking cessation in South Asian communities

Q Zaidi

Introduction

Tobacco smoking is a well established risk factor for CHD. In subgroups of the South Asian populations, the prevalence of smoking habits varies significantly. South Asian females rarely smoke in these populations (or at least rarely report smoking, though this is changing in the younger South Asians), whereas the prevalence of smoking in males varies according to ethnic subgroup (Table 10.1) e.g. in the Health Survey for England '99[1], 44% of Bangladeshi males smoked compared to 23% of Indian males, the latter reflecting more closely the prevalence of smoking in the general population. Within South Asian communities, there is a link between the observed rates of smoking and socio-economic deprivation. Higher rates of smoking in certain groups can also be attributed to the 'social acceptance' of smoking[2]. It has been argued that the heterogeneity of South Asian populations is an important consideration in developing health programmes[3]. Many health professionals regard South Asians as one community. However there are many differences between individual groups in terms of religion, customs, traditions, languages, education, and economic status. Their attitudes and beliefs about health and disease also differ. Therefore, in designing smoking cessation programmes for South Asians this heterogeneity should be taken into account. In addition, the 'chewing' of tobacco and related products is common in certain South Asian communities, particularly the Bangladeshi community, in both males and females.

This chapter will focus on smoking cessation behaviour in South Asian communities, examining the impact of national initiatives on smoking prevalence in these communities. The chapter will also highlight the reasons why these communities need specific targeting and innovative approaches to reduce smoking.

Table 10.1 Smoking and quitting rates for South Asian groups, compared to the general population. Extracted from the Health Survey for England 1999[1]

	Males				Females	
	Smoking	Chewing	Quit attempt	Quit success	Smoking	Chewing
Indian	23%	2%	61%	35%	6%	6%
Pakistani	26%	2%	55%	21%	5%	6%
Bangladeshi	44%	19%	71%	19%	1%	26%
General Population	27%	NS	>70%	54%	27%	NS

NS (not stated)

Government Initiatives

Following the 1998 White Paper on smoking[4] the government has undertaken several national initiatives. The major achievements as result of this paper have been the establishment of specialist smoking cessation services in every primary care trust and the availability of nicotine replacement therapy (NRT) and bupropion (Zyban) on prescription to those patients deemed ready for smoking cessation.

Quitting smoking amongst South Asians

Table 10.1 shows that in terms of attempts at quitting, the intention of South Asian male smokers to give up is similar to the general population. However, actual quit rates are much lower than in the general, predominantly white population and the utilisation of services designed to help people give up smoking is lower in South Asian populations. Most smoking cessation services have failed to attract ethnic minority groups. However services designed specifically for ethnic groups such as those in Coventry, Bradford, Camden and East London, have attracted fairly large numbers of Asian smokers. This suggests that service adaptations are necessary for addressing the needs of South Asian smokers. The justification for programmes specifically targeted to particular groups takes into account the higher prevalence of smoking of Bangladeshis and the fact that there are language and cultural barriers inhibiting smokers from many ethnic minority groups from joining specialist clinics.

Reasons why quitting rates are lower amongst South Asians

To see how we should address the problem of lower quit rates amongst South Asian groups, one needs to identify the reasons for this phenomenon. Bush *et al*[2] pointed out that the social acceptability of smoking in Pakistani and Bangladeshi communities might contribute to a lower quit rate. In our experience at the BHF we have found the following reasons for lower quit rates

- A low level of awareness amongst South Asians of the health risks associated with smoking.
- Low awareness of the addictiveness of cigarettes.
- Very little awareness of the availability of NRT and bupropion, and of their effectiveness.
- A social acceptability of smoking in some Asian groups.
- Fatalistic attitudes to health.
- Perception of a lack of control over health.
- Low self esteem.
- Poor socio-economic conditions.

According to the, 'Black and Minority Ethnic Groups in England, the second lifestyle survey (2000)', South Asians' knowledge of the health risks of smoking is poor[5]. Only 25% of South Asians perceive there to be a link between cigarette smoking and heart disease. This knowledge decreased with increasing age.

The British Heart Foundation strategy

Where attempts are made to quit smoking, outcomes are not as successful as for the general population (data drawn from HEA 2000). Consequently a three-step approach to reduce the prevalence of smoking is advocated by the British Heart Foundation (BHF). The first step is to bridge the knowledge gap. The BHF recommend the use of the media, places of worship and social networks. The second step is to ensure that the community feels empowered to make positive lifestyle changes and for this, community involvement and a developmental approach is required. An 'attitude and norm change' strategy would assist in reducing smoking. Campaigns to reduce exposure to second hand smoking at home and the workplace would also help. Thirdly, the variety of methods available to quit smoking need to be widely applied. The BHF policy calls for actions to facilitate this three-step approach, in particular ensuring that the knowledge gap is addressed and available services are promoted.

Bridging the knowledge gap

In 2002 just prior to the national 'No Smoking Day' the BHF conducted a small survey of knowledge about NRT and bupropion at Asian Quitline and found that only 3 callers out of a poll of 100 knew about Zyban and only 6 had heard about NRT. Most callers were unaware that these aids could potentially double their chances of quitting. Unless this gap in knowledge and awareness about smoking cessation aids is addressed it is unlikely that one will witness an increase the number of quitters from South Asian communities. It is noteworthy that many Asians in deprived inner city areas are registered with 'single handed practices', where general practitioners may not have time to give detailed advice about smoking cessation. Asian Quitline has also noted that where patients have had cardiac surgery or myocardial infarction, they are rarely informed about NRT or bupropion. GPs surgeries can, however, be used by advisors to give information on quitting. It has been found that opportunistic health education, provided to members of ethnic minorities, at the time of clinic attendance, has been well received by both sexes[6].

To bridge this knowledge gap Asian media can play a central role. At Asian Quitline the number of calls are significantly increased when media campaigns using popular

South Asian media are undertaken. There is also anecdotal evidence that first generation Asians prefer such media and tend to watch South Asian TV channels more than mainstream channels.

To overcome the difficulties of reaching minority ethnic groups many health promoters have started to train community workers in health issues in the hope that they may pass on information to others. There are examples of health promotion services running courses for community workers covering diverse health issues (e.g. Project Dil 2002 in Leicester). Furthermore many primary care trusts have trained smoking advisors who are working with ethnic minority groups (Camden PCT 2002). Smoking guidelines[7] have suggested and reinforced this practice of the use of paid trained community workers.

To increase the awareness of dangers of smoking and available methods of quitting, places of worship can also play a major role. On important religious festivals, large mosques, gurudwaras and mandirs can attract thousands of people and with the help of these institutions health promoters can reach significant numbers within these communities.

The BHF have been funding Asian Quitline since 1997 to provide culturally appropriate telephone counselling and support service to those smokers who wish to quit smoking. Asian Quitline has also been involved in outreach work, in which it has been working with community groups, places of worship and has been involved in training of health professionals to equip them to deliver culturally sensitive smoking cessation programmes in the community. For the past five years Asian Quitline have been running a Ramadan campaign. In this campaign mosques in the UK are targeted using Imams who have been trained in giving basic smoking cessation advice. Furthermore, trained lay smoking advisors are also used to provide one-to-one information to interested groups.

Community empowerment

Providing information is not sufficient. Although understanding a health issue may be a necessary precursor to action, it is certainly not sufficient. It should be accompanied by a process of belief and values-clarification which should be followed by some practice in decision making and this would increase the capacity to freely choose from various alternatives. Bhopal & White[8] have argued that skills and confidence to change behaviour are more important than knowledge. This process increases the self-esteem of participants, particularly those with low self-esteem, who are unlikely to look after themselves. It has been mentioned that contrary to popular opinion older South Asians feel lonely and isolated which may lead to low self esteem[9]. This may also reduce the probability of quitting smoking. Therefore individual and community empowerment would lead to higher smoking cessation rates.

Bush *et al*[2] have found that smoking among Pakistani and Bangladeshi men is seen as socially acceptable and, not surprisingly we see higher levels of smoking among them. In contrast smoking in women in these groups is stigmatised and not acceptable, hence there is a low rate of smoking among women. Therefore, one must work to change prevailing norms and attitudes within minority ethnic societies. This can only be achieved by working with social, community and religious leaders. Hopefully, this may create an environment where smoking is generally viewed as being 'socially unacceptable'. 'Denormalisation' is based on the notion of changing social norms. The social norm change model is based on the fact that the thoughts, values and actions of individuals are tempered by their community[10]

Within the individual household setting one will also need to raise awareness of the harmful effects of second-hand tobacco smoke. Here one may work with young people and have them encourage parents, relatives and visitors not to smoke at home.

Relative merits of methods for quitting smoking

According to the Government White Paper on Tobacco (1998), 'a full course of specialist counselling combined with NRT can lead up to 25% of smokers to give up'. There is strong evidence of the effectiveness of NRT (in the form of chewing gum, transdermal patch, nasal spray, inhaler, tablet or lozenge) in assisting smoking cessation for nicotine dependant smokers. This intervention increased the chances of smoking cessation by one and a half to two times[7]. However, all trials combined NRT with at least brief advice, and the quit rate was higher when NRT was combined with intensive support. There is, therefore, a strong argument for the use of brief advice to be offered as a minimum in support of NRT (National Electronic Library for health and heart disease website: 'Which interventions are most effective' and National Institute for Clinical Excellence[11]). According to the National Service Framework (NSF) for coronary heart disease[12], studies from the United States of America suggest that smoking cessation interventions with black and minority ethnic groups can be effective. The NSF (2000) also states:

- Literature should be multi-lingual and in a culturally appropriate style.
- Communications campaigns should be used to redress misperceptions about tobacco use.
- Ethnic differences in terms of attitudes and beliefs towards tobacco should be incorporated into smoking cessation interventions.

Conclusion

Smoking prevalence in the most economically deprived South Asian communities is higher than in the general population, but desire to quit in these communities is similar to that in the general population. However due to cultural acceptance of smoking and lack of awareness of smoking cessation aids, language and cultural barriers, cessation rates are lower than general population. To decrease smoking prevalence and encourage smokers to quit we need a comprehensive strategy which South Asian media, social and religious leaders and social networks could use to change norms to make smoking socially unacceptable. Help and support tailored to their needs, should be provided to those who wish to quit. A grass roots approach is required to reduce smoking prevalence in South Asian communities.

References

1.   Joint health services unit. Health Survey for England. The health of minority ethnic groups' 99. London, The stationery office, 2001.

2.   Bush, J., White M., Kai, J., Rankin, J., and Bhopal, R., Smoking in Bangladeshi and Pakistani adults: community based, qualitative study BMJ 2003, 326: 962.

3.   Bhopal R, Unwin N, White M, Yallop J, Walker L, Alberti KJMM, et al Heterogeneity of coronary heart disease risk factors in Indian, Pakistani, Bangladeshi, and European origin populations: cross sectional study. BMJ 1999:319:215-220

4.   Department of Health. Smoking Kills, white paper on tobacco, London. HMSO, 1998a.

5.   Johnson MR, Owen D, Blackburn C (2000). Black & ethnic minority groups in England: the second health & lifestyles survey. London: Health education Authority.

6.   Hawthorne K. Diabetes health education for British South Asians: a review of aims, difficulties and achievements. Health Education Journal 1994: 53: 309-321.

7.   West R, McNeill A, Raw M. Smoking cessation guidelines for health professionals: an update. Thorax 2000: 55:987-999.

8.   Bhopal RS, White M. Health promotion for ethnic minorities: past, present and future. In: Ahmed WIU (editor). 'Race' and health in contemporary Britain. Milton Keynes: Open University Press, 1993.

9.   Modood, T. Changing ethnic identities. Policy Studies Institute PSI, London, 1994.

10.   A model for change: The Californian experience in tobacco control. Californian Dept. of Health Services Tobacco Control Section, Oct. 1998.

11.   National Institute for Clinical Excellence. Guidance on the use of nicotine replacement therapy (NRT) and bupropion for smoking cessation. March 2002

12.   Department of Health. National Service Framework on Coronary Heart Disease. London; Chapter 1 – Reducing Heart Disease in the Population, 2000. P9

11

Physical activity among South Asians in Britain

M White

Introduction

Physical inactivity is an established independent risk factor for CHD, diabetes, stroke, hypertension, obesity and osteoporosis[1]. It is also thought to be important in promoting mental health[2]. Physical activity has direct, positive effects on cardiovascular and respiratory systems, and on glucose and lipid metabolism. However, these positive effects are short-lived and lost once regular activity ceases. In other words, only regular physical activity is truly beneficial.[1]

A detailed understanding of the experience of physical activity among South Asian communities is essential to underpin the development of effective interventions to promote regular exercise. This paper sets out to answer a number of questions pertinent to this challenge:

- How inactive are South Asian males and females?
- Are there generational differences?
- How good is their knowledge of the benefits of regular activity?
- What are their attitudes to physical activity?
- Are their reasons for inactivity specific to South Asian communities?
- What can be done to promote physical activity in South Asian communities

In reviewing physical activity among South Asians, I have drawn on the work of a limited number of authors. Although these do represent the main work on this topic, it is important to stress that this is not a systematic review. Our work on the epidemiology of cardiovascular diseases and diabetes among South Asians has demonstrated the importance of studying distinct ethnic sub-groups within the South Asian population[3]. Thus a key criterion for choosing studies was their ability to distinguish between Indians, Pakistanis and Bangladeshis. The studies I have reviewed are as follows:

1. The Health Survey for England '99[4]. This biennial national survey used questions originally derived from the Allied Dunbar National Fitness Survey[5] and, in 1999, had a particular focus on ethnic minority groups, with a sample boosted to represent the main ethnic groups in England. It provides descriptive epidemiological data on level and intensity of activity, but little explanatory analysis and no qualitative data.

2. The Health Education Authority (HEA) 2nd health and lifestyles survey of black and ethnic minority groups in England, 1994[6]. This representative population survey focused on ethnic minority groups and, as well as collecting data on levels of activity, asked about types of activity, opportunities and barriers to activity, and knowledge and attitudes.

3. The National Study of Health & Growth[7]. This is the only study of health related behaviours among children that reports data specifically on ethnic minority groups. However, South Asians are not distinguished by ethnic sub-group.

4. The Newcastle Heart Project, 1995-7[3, 8, 9]. Although a local epidemiological study, this study has a geographically representative population coverage and detailed data on both health behaviours and health states, including cardiovascular disease.

How inactive are South Asian males and females?

In the Health Survey for England[4], there was an ethnic gradient in participation in sports and recreational exercise among adults, with highest levels in the general, predominantly white population, followed by Indians, then Pakistanis, with the lowest levels in Bangladeshi males and females. Males were more likely to engage in regular sports and heavy manual or 'DIY' activities than females. Significantly fewer males, however, undertook regular, heavy housework, and this pattern was the same in all ethnic groups. There was also an ethnic gradient in brisk walking in both males and females, with highest levels in the general population and lowest in Bangladeshis (Figure 11.1).

Figure 11.1: Participation in physical activity in previous 4 weeks by ethnic group[4]

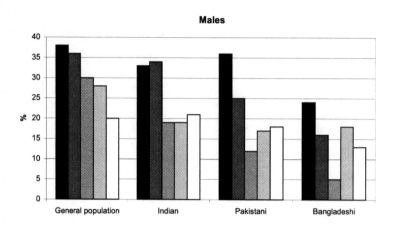

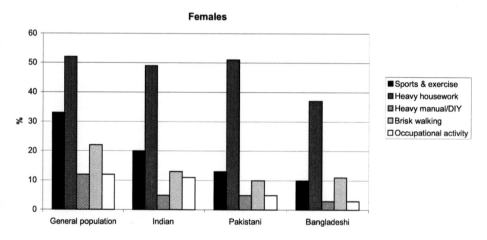

In the Newcastle Heart Project, there were similar ethnic gradients for achievement of national physical activity targets (at least 30 minutes of at least moderate activity on 5 days of the week[10]) among adults aged 25-74 years, with European origin study participants most active and Bangladeshis least active and, apart from among Pakistanis, males being more active than females. However, even among European males (the most active group), only 48% were achieving this target level; among Bangladeshi females (the least active group), only 9% achieved this target. With regard to vigorous activity, only 1% of Bangladeshi females are regularly active, compared with 26% of males and females in the general population[4].

Are there generational differences?

In the national data, there was a strong age gradient, with lowest levels of activity in those aged over 55 years in all ethnic groups, suggesting there is no ethnic group specific generational effect[4]. However, perhaps more worrying, in their National Study of Health & Growth, Bettiol *et al* showed that, in comparison with White and Afro-Caribbean 8-9 year olds, three times as many children of families from the Indian sub-continent (India, Pakistan and Bangladesh) were unable to complete a cycle ergometer test (to 85% of maximum heart rate) for physical fitness[7]. Whilst the authors acknowledge that there may be some bias, resulting from unfamiliarity with a bicycle among the Asian children, it is unlikely to have accounted for such a large difference in fitness.

In summary, South Asians adults in Britain are generally less active than Europeans, both in terms of participation in sports and in 'lifestyle' activity. Among South Asians, Bangladeshis are least active and Indians most active. Studies of children show South Asians to be less active and less fit than European children. To explore further the possible reasons for these findings, I have looked at data on attitudes to, and knowledge of, physical activity.

How good is knowledge of the benefits of regular activity within South Asian communities?

In the HEA's Black and Minority Ethnic Groups survey, South Asian adults were asked: *"What serious illness or health problems are linked to not taking enough exercise?"*. The most commonly mentioned problems were 'being overweight' (41% overall, with little ethnic difference), 'heart disease' (32% of Indian and Pakistanis, 17% of Bangladeshis); 'joint problems' (11% overall, with little ethnic difference); and 'diabetes' and 'stroke' (6% overall, with little ethnic variation). Perhaps more worrying was the fact that around 20% of Indian males and females and Pakistani females did not know of any related health problems, whereas 26% of Bangladeshi males, 29% of Pakistani females and 38% of Bangladeshi females knew of no health problems associated with lack of activity[6]. Given the rapid current growth of chronic diseases among South Asian ethnic groups, especially Bangladeshis and Pakistanis[3], this is a worrying deficit in important risk-related knowledge.

In summary, knowledge of physical activity reflect gradients in activity: Bangladeshis appear least knowledgeable compared with Pakistanis and Indians.

What are the prevailing attitudes to physical activity among South Asian communities?

The HEA's Black and Minority Ethnic Groups survey explored attitudes and knowledge of physical activity. Pakistani and Bangladeshi females, who have the lowest levels of activity, reported the key reasons[6] for non-participation in recreational activities as:

'looking after young children' (29%)
'insufficient time' (26%);
'won't go to mixed-sex facilities' (20%);
'won't go to places where people show parts of their bodies' (19%);
'fear of going out alone' (17%).

Language and culture were otherwise rarely mentioned and it is important to emphasise that 40% of females and 70% of males said none of the listed 'ethnic group specific' reasons for inactivity applied to them.

Ethnically specific factors affecting participation in physical activity are more prevalent among Pakistanis and Bangladeshis, especially females, but overall, these may not be the most important factors determining physical activity among South Asian groups.

Are their other reasons for inactivity, specific to South Asian communities?

One important factor relating to the social context of South Asian families in the UK is their relative economic position. This has been explored in relation to cardiovascular disease[9] as well as other health states[11], and it is widely recognised that a socio-economic gradient exists, with Bangladeshis having the lowest incomes and social status in the UK, followed by Pakistanis, with Indians enjoying a socio-economic status almost equivalent to the general population[11]. The relationship between social class, ethnicity and participation in activity was explored in the National Health Survey for England (Figure 11.2). The pattern is somewhat curious.

Figure 11.2: Participation in vigorous activity for 30 minutes on 5 or more days/week, by social class, ethnicity and sex

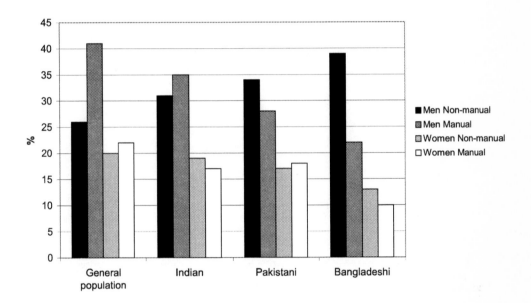

Although the ethnic trends are as expected for males and females from manual social classes, and for females from non-manual social classes, the trend is reversed for males in the non manual social class group, indicating that Bangladeshi professionals and managers are more likely to take regular vigorous activity than those from other ethnic groups. Thus we can see that among the general population and Indians, males in manual social classes were more likely to be vigorously active than males in non-manual social classes. The same effect was seen for females among the general population. These patterns may, in part, be related to different patterns of occupations among the different groups, and thus seen as part of a more general pattern of socio-economic transition among these ethnic minority populations. Occupations, income and social status are known to play important roles in determining levels of physical activity in the general population and may also have specific effects among South Asian communities.

What can be done to promote physical activity in South Asian communities?

There is little evidence to support the implementation of interventions to promote physical activity among South Asian communities[8, 12]. The evidence base to support interventions in the general population is also weak and few interventions have been shown to have long term effectiveness[13]. Some interventions have been tested among South Asian groups (e.g. Muslim females[12]), but no objective outcome evaluations have been reported as yet. Until a stronger and more specific evidence base is available, efforts to promote physical activity among South Asian communities should be based on the best available evidence from the general population, applied as appropriate within South Asian communities using the principles recommended by the HEA and others to guide health promotion among ethnic minority groups[14, 15].

Conclusions

We do not know enough about the reasons why South Asians are so inactive, nor what would help to promote greater activity. Greater understanding requires further research. Studies are needed to monitor activity and fitness in successive cohorts of South Asian children and adults in order to identify emerging trends. Detailed qualitative research will help us to understand better the barriers to and opportunities for physical activity, and develop culturally acceptable interventions. These will then need to be tested for efficacy and effectiveness in appropriate outcome evaluations within South Asian communities. Developments in practice need to be across a range of sectors, including local leisure services, transport, education and the health service.

Acknowledgements

Many people contributed to our research on South Asians in Newcastle and they are acknowledged in Reference 3 below. Raj Bhopal and Louise Hayes in particular provided helpful advice and support on work discussed in this paper.

References

1. Fentem PH (1991). Benefits of exercise in health and disease. BMJ; 308:1291-5.

2. Mutrie N, Biddle SJH (1995). The effects of exercise on mental health in clinical populations. In: Biddle SJH (editor). European perspectives on exercise and sports psychology. Leeds: Humana Kinetics, 1995.

3. Bhopal R, Unwin N, White M, et al (1999). Heterogeneity in coronary heart disease and risk factors in Indian, Pakistani, Bangladeshi and European origin populations. BMJ; 319: 215-220.

4. Erens B, Primatesta P, Prior PE (2000). Health Survey for England. The health of ethnic groups 1999. London: Department of Health.

5. HEA/Sports Council (1992). Allied Dunbar National Fitness Survey: Main Findings. London: HEA/Sports Council.

6. Johnson MR, Owen D, Blackburn C (2000). Black & ethnic minority groups in England: the second health & lifestyles survey. London: Health education Authority.

7. Bettiol H, Rona RJ, Chinn S, (1999). Variation in physical fitness between ethnic groups in nine-year olds. Int. J Epidemiol; 28: 281-6.

8. Hayes L, White M, Bhopal RS, et al (2002). Patterns of physical activity and relationship with risk markers for cardiovascular disease and diabetes in Indian, Pakistani, Bangladeshi and European adults in a UK population. J Public Health Med; 24: 170-8.

9. Bhopal RS, Hayes L, White M, et al (2002). Ethnic and socio-economic inequalities in coronary heart disease, diabetes and risk factors in European and South Asian. J Public Health Med; 24: 95-105.

10. Pate RR, Pratt M, Blair SN, et al (1995). Physical Activity and Public Health: A recommendation from the Centers for Disease Control and the American College of Sports Medicine. JAMA 273(5): 402-407.

11. Nazroo J (1997). The health of Britain's ethnic minorities. London: Policy Studies Institute.

12.   Carroll R, Ali N, Azam N. (2002). Promoting physical activity in South Asian Muslim females through 'exercise on prescription.' Health technology Assessment; 6(8).

13.   Hillsdon M., Foster C, et al. (2002). Interventions for Promoting Physical Activity. The Cochrane Database of Systematic Reviews. 2002.

14.   Sahrif S (1997). Active for life. Guidelines for promoting physical activity with black and minority ethnic groups. London: Health Education Authority.

15.   Bhopal RS, White M (1993). Health promotion for ethnic minorities: past, present and future. In: Ahmed WIU (editor). 'Race' and health in contemporary Britain. Milton Keynes: Open University Press.

12

Poverty, stress and racism as factors in South Asian heart disease

R Williams and S Harding

Introduction

Complementary to reviews of physiological and genetic causes of South Asian heart disease, we aim to discuss three important social factors, not necessarily to provide an alternative explanation, but more probably as a deeper background influence which may be affecting a number of physiological pathways. It is important to recognise that the strength of a social influence is not limited to any particular physiological pathway with which it is linked, but is usually the sum of various scattered pathways, both known and unknown. This summary will focus on recent research which has explicitly sought to link at least one of these social factors with an accepted pathway of risk for heart disease.

Research on poverty, stress, and racism as factors in heart disease has had a curious development shaped by the political history of the last five decades. From the 1960s to the 1980s, poverty and racism were researched as social issues, primarily in the UK and USA. The civil rights movement in the USA, centred on Black Americans, roused echoes in the UK as another Anglophone country with a black population in deprived circumstances. The research was primarily sociological, and the South Asian communities were included only as another group which could fall under a politicised Black label. At the same time research was developing on South Asian heart disease as a separate issue, mostly centred in different locations which included the UK, Trinidad, Malaysia and South Africa, destinations of South Asian migrants under the former British Empire. This research was primarily clinical and epidemiological.

The connection between these two lines of research had common geographical ground only in the UK, and as a result the question whether poverty, stress and racism had a connection with South Asian heart disease was to become primarily a UK question. And at first, on the data available in the 1960s to the 1980s, it seemed that it was a question destined to be answered "no". Taking poverty first, no social class gradient was found in South Asian CHD mortality in the first study linking mortality with country of birth on data from 1970-78[1]. When consideration moved to stress, the principal review of the situation published in 1989[2] found no evidence of higher levels of psychiatric distress in South Asians in the research conducted up to that time, mainly in Birmingham. As for racism, the main obstacle to confirming a link was the absence of any evidence of excess CHD in the UK Black Caribbean population, which was taken to be the paradigmatic case for experience of racism. It was soon suggested, though, that there might be different physiological pathways which explained the high South Asian CHD rates and the high incidence of stroke in Black Caribbeans as responses to the same stressors[1].

If there was in fact a connection, therefore, between excess South Asian CHD and poverty, stress and racism, it was going to be a matter of penetrating disguises which had cloaked this link in preceding data, and the research of the 1990s set out to examine this possibility.

The re-emerging social class gradient

The first of these disguises to be penetrated was the absence of a social class gradient in South Asian heart disease. Research in the Medical Research Council (MRC) Medical Sociology Unit programme indicated that there had been a temporary disruption of class chances and standard of living gradients in the South Asian population in the period after their migration[3]. By class chances is meant the link between occupational level and standard of living – this was broken because South Asians entered the UK labour force at quite different levels to those which they had held in the economy of the subcontinent, and had very varying success in re-establishing a stable connection between their qualifications and their occupational level. Many well-educated people sank, and many shrewd and energetic people overcame educational deficits to prosper in their own business enterprises. By standard of living gradients is meant the link between standard of living and mortality or morbidity – because standard of living was so variable in these conditions, no stable connection could be discerned for some decades.

However by 1987 standard of living gradients were re-emerging, at least in CHD risk behaviours, though it was likely that this would take time to work through into chronic morbidity and mortality[3]. By 1993/4, standard of living gradients were confirmed in South Asian reports of CHD, with more than half of the excess reported by Pakistanis and Bangladeshis being accounted for in this way[4,5]. In the 1991-3 mortality data a social class gradient in South Asian CHD had also re-emerged[6].

In the last three years, a burst of activity has added detail to these findings. In the Whitehall study of UK civil servants, adjusting for socio-economic grade (probably a finer index of standard of living in this setting than social class position) attenuates excess biochemical CHD risk in South Asian civil servants, though it does not abolish it[7]. Similarly in data from the 1991 UK Census with deaths from 1991-3, adjusting for social class gradients attenuates, though it does not explain, Pakistani and Bangladeshi CHD mortality (until social class position is securely linked with standard of living in South Asian families who are self-employed attenuation can be expected to be incomplete)[8]. A retrospective look at the UK ONS Longitudinal Study, which began in 1971, reveals that social class and deprivation gradients began to emerge in South Asian mortality generally during the period after 1981 up to 1997[9]. At a finer-grain level, it appears from the 1993-7 Newcastle study that the socio-economic gradient was then strongest in CHD risk behaviours, and in the longest-resident subgroup (Indians), and was still uncertain in biochemical measures and in other groups[10].

Re-assessing stress and racism

Stress is often a vague term, but four quite specific psychosocial determinants of CHD have been confirmed in numerous previous prospective cohort studies[11]:

1. Anxiety and depression
2. Hostility and Type A personality
3. Particular kinds of job strain

4. Low social support

These determinants may affect CHD directly or work through health behaviour. At the same time they may themselves be the outcome either of low socio-economic position, or of racism. A resulting model can be formulated as in Figure 12.1.

Figure 12.1. A model to explain the psychosocial determinants of CHD (SES=socioecomonic status)

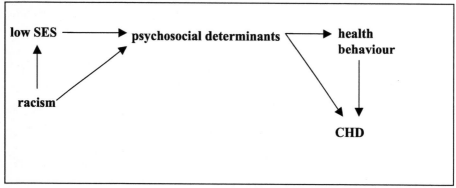

We noted earlier that at first little evidence was found of excess anxiety and depression amongst South Asians; hence if excess levels were in fact disguised, the question had to be whether there was some form of denial in habitual modes of expressing psychological distress. This possibility was accentuated by research on Black Americans in the 1990s. Blood pressure in this group was found to be higher in those who said they had experienced no racism[12], or in those claiming least experience of racism as well as those claiming most such experience[13]. It was also higher in those who said they would say nothing and do nothing about racist incidents. In addition Black Americans had also been found by Dressler during the 1980s to manifest a characteristic psychosomatic expression of distress[14].

Amongst South Asians, the possibility seemed to be that anxiety and depression are somatised. Dressler's psychosomatic measure was used in the MRC's 1987 data referred to earlier, and was found to be sensitive to experience of poverty, stress in work about the house, and experience of assault (including racist assaults), while psychological distress as measured by the General Health Questionnaire (GHQ) remained insensitive[15]. The GHQ is a standard, well-attested screening measure of expressed distress in the UK population and many others[16]. There are indications, however, that the language in which distress is expressed is important. Self-assessed distress on a very simple verbal measure was just as sensitive to factors affecting the psychosomatic measure in the MRC data. South Asian women, Muslims and limited English speakers all showed excess distress on these more sensitive measures, and the poverty and stress measures were sufficient to explain this distress. At the same time, the GHQ is in fact sensitive to South Asian experience of stress in paid work[15]. In the Whitehall study, South Asian civil servants were more depressed than white civil servants on this measure[17].

Turning to hostility, and the frustrations associated in early research with what was called the Type A personality, it has been found that hostility is related to high effort and low reward, and this combination in turn predicts CHD[18]. Recently the Whitehall study has shown that South Asian civil servants experience more effort/reward imbalance, and have higher hostility levels, than white civil servants[17]. A link of this kind may well underlie the allied finding in the ONS Longitudinal Study that downward job mobility predicts a higher risk of limiting longstanding illness in South Asians and West Indians than in other members of the study[19]. This being so, further research is also needed on another characteristic occupational niche of South Asians in Britain – the low-income, self-employed situation, where high effort and low reward are only too likely concomitants.

Job strain has increasingly been linked with low job control. In the UK civil service, South Asians have less job control than whites, and this is explained by the fact that they have lower job grades. However, at each job grade, South Asians have higher educational qualifications than whites[17].

Social support has a number of dimensions, and the picture is usually a balance of opposing tendencies. More South Asians of the migrant generation are married than the general population of the same age; however more see parents and siblings less than once a year, and more South Asian women have no parents or siblings nearby (a feature of the patrilocal tendency which constructs households around husbands and their fathers). As a result of this combination of familial and migratory patterns, fewer South Asian migrants than the general population in Britain say they have "someone to turn to when something is bothering them or they are feeling low"[20]; and those with no one to turn to are more likely to be distressed[15]. These patterns are likely to change in the UK-born generation, where more households are located near the wife's parents. There is also the question of whether social relationships are positive or negative for the parties concerned. In the Whitehall study South Asian civil servants more often had negative social relationships (though men had more confiding support). They also had less social support at work[17].

In all four dimensions of psychosocial risk for CHD, therefore, South Asians are now emerging as at high risk. The time is at hand to test systematically for the extent to which these results are linked with poverty and racism, as in the model set out in Figure 12.1. Meanwhile this model can be further expanded to include the question whether South Asians with potential CHD-related symptoms are able to get adequate health care.

Access of CHD patients to proper health care

Racism is a spectrum of behaviour in which frank, overt, intentional racism is not a very common component, at least in the UK. More common is covert antagonistic behaviour, or routine behaviour of a kind which puts members of particular cultural minorities at a disadvantage because the actor has not thought about possible consequences in that context. An expanded model would acknowledge that poverty and racism are both capable of reducing chances of access to good health care, and this in turn could affect CHD survival, as in Figure 12.2.

Figure 12.2. A hypothetical model to link poverty and racism to CHD

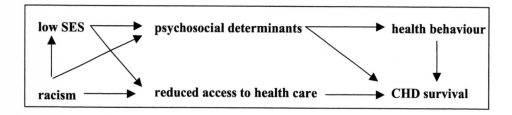

A number of studies suggest that obstacles to care of heart disease which fall under the broad heading of racism, as defined above, are in fact occurring. Back in 1993, time from onset of angina symptoms until referral to a regional cardiothoracic centre was found to be ten months longer in Indian origin patients than in European patients matched for age, sex and extent of coronary disease[21]. This raises the question whether the reason for this is likely to be in the patient's illness behaviour – the interpretation of symptoms, for example – or in the clinician's response. A subsequent study in London found that Hindus and Sikhs actually report greater likelihood of seeking immediate care for angina symptoms than Europeans[22]. This placed the onus of investigation on the clinician. Already in 1989, it had been reported that native British patients were more likely to leave their GP surgery with a follow-up appointment [23]. Follow-up studies of such patterns are now a matter of urgency.

Conclusion

In the matter of whether poverty, stress and racism are contributing to excess South Asian heart disease, science has now come full circle. What seemed an implausible hypothesis in the 1960s-1980s now seems, after careful detective work which has penetrated many disguises, a hypothesis which is overdue for re-testing. The model developed in Figure 2 provides a basis for research in the first decade of the new millennium. This research needs to identify prospective cohorts on a national scale, and to integrate the piecemeal advances of the 1990s by systematic tests on all the linkages outlined in the model. This is a hypothesis which will run and run.

References

1.   Marmot M, Adelstein A, Bulusu L. Immigrant mortality in England and Wales 1970-78: causes of death by country of birth. London: HMSO; 1984.

2.   McKeigue PM, Miller GJ, Marmot MG. Coronary heart disease in South Asians overseas: a review. Journal Clinical Epidemiology 1989;42(7):597-609.

3.   Williams R, Wright W, Hunt K. Social class and health: the puzzling counter-example of British South Asians. Social Science and Medicine 1998;47(9):1277-1288.

4.   Nazroo JY. The health of Britain's ethnic minorities. Findings from a national survey. London: Policy Studies Institute; 1997.

5.   Nazroo JY. South Asian people and heart disease: an assessment of the importance of socioeconomic position. Ethnicity and Disease 2001;11:401-411.

6.   Harding S, Maxwell R. Differences in mortality of migrants. In: Drever F, Whitehead M, editors. Health inequalities: decennial supplement. London: The Stationery Office; 1997.

7.   Whitty CJM, Brunner EJ, Shipley MJ, Hemingway H, Marmot MG. Differences in biological risk factors for cardiovascular disease between three ethnic groups in the Whitehall II study. Atherosclerosis 1999;142:279-286.

8.   Harding S. Examining the contribution to high cardiovascular mortality among Indian, Pakistani and Bangladeshi male immigrants living in England and Wales. Health Statistics Quarterly 2000;5:26-28.

9.   Harding S, Balarajan R. Longitudinal study of socio-economic differences in mortality among South Asian and West Indian migrants. Ethnicity & Health 2001;6(2):121-128.

10.   Bhopal R, Hayes L, White M, Unwin N, Harland J, Ayis S, et al. Ethnic and socio-economic inequalities in coronary heart disease, diabetes and risk factors in Europeans and South Asians. Journal of Public Health Medicine 2002;24(2):95-105.

11.   Hemingway H, Marmot MG. Psychosocial factors in the aetiology and prognosis of coronary heart disease: a systematic review of prospective cohort studies. British Medical Journal 1999;318:1460-1467.

12.   Krieger N. Racial and gender discrimination: risk factors for high blood pressure? Social Science and Medicine 1990;30(12):1273-1281.

13.   Krieger N, Sidney S. Racial discrimination and blood pressure: the CARDIA study of young black and white adults. American Journal of Public Health 1996;86(10):1370-1378.

14.   Dressler WW. Psychosomatic symptoms, stress and modernization: a model. Culture, Medicine and Psychiatry 1985;9:257-286.

15.   Williams R, Hunt K. Psychological distress among British South Asians: the contribution of stressful situations and subcultural differences in the West of Scotland Twenty-07 Study. Psychological Medicine 1997;27:1173-1181.

16.   Goldberg DP. The detection of psychiatric illness by questionnaire. Oxford: Oxford University Press; 1972.

17.   Hemingway H, Whitty C, Shipley M, Stansfeld S, Brunner E, Marmot M. Psychosocial risk factors for coronary disease in white, South Asian and Afro-Caribbean civil servants: the Whitehall II Study. Ethnicity and Disease 2001;11:391-400.

18.   Bosma H, Peter R, Siegrist J, Marmot MG. Two alternative job stress models and the risk of coronary heart disease. American Journal of Public Health 1998;88:68-74.

19.   Harding S. Social mobility and self-reported limiting long-term illness among West Indian and South Asian migrants living in England and Wales. Social Science and Medicine 2003; 56: 355-361.

20.   Williams R, Bhopal R, Hunt K. Coronary risk in a British Punjabi population: comparative profile of non-biochemical factors. International Journal of Epidemiology 1994;23(1):28-37.

21.   Shaukat N, de Bono DP, Cruickshank JK. Clinical features, risk factors, and referral delay in British patients of Indian and European origin with angina matched for age and extent of coronary atheroma. British Medical Journal 1993;307:717-718.

22.   Chaturvedi N, Rai H, Ben-Shlomo Y. Lay diagnosis and health-care-seeking behaviour for chest pain in south Asians and Europeans. The Lancet 1997;350:1578-1583.

23.   Gillam S, Jarman B, White P, Law R. Ethnic differences in consultation rates in urban general practice. British Medical Journal 1989;299:953-957.

13

Overview of South Asian coronary heart disease and the road ahead

M Marmot

The high rate of coronary heart disease (CHD) in South Asians has attracted high quality research. It is well represented in the chapters of this book. There are at least three reasons why research in this area is timely and much needed. First, there is the problem itself. To take action to reduce this health burden, proper scientific understanding is necessary. Research findings should guide intervention efforts. Second, understanding this particular problem has the potential for shedding light on areas of the causes of CHD that are imperfectly understood. Examining ethnic differences in disease is a way of testing older hypotheses and developing and refining new ones. Third, research in this area has much to teach on approaches to understanding and researching ethnic differences in disease.

It is, unfortunately, quite common in research to have a great deal of data but few ideas. In this area ideas abound; it is the data that are lacking. There are, for example, clear hints that CHD rates are higher in urban areas in India than in rural areas, but few data that document this clearly or shed light on why it should be the case. Similarly, there are interesting suggestions that coronary risk factors are elevated among UK South Asian men compared to their brothers in India who did not migrate. Systematic investigation of migrants has great potential to illuminate how genetic predisposition may interact with environmental and lifestyle changes. There are a number of competing explanations for the high rate of CHD in South Asians, but the lack of a cohort study of sufficient power to investigate the causes of ethnic variations in CHD.

In the absence of such data, it is reasonable to assume that risk factors, established as such in other populations, will also predict disease in South Asians. Knowing that a risk factor is predictive in South Asians does not, by itself, account for the excess CHD in South Asians. For example, LDL cholesterol and smoking are lower in some South Asian groups than in the general population in England[1]. We must look elsewhere for explanations.

The studies that McKeigue[2] and I did pointed to the potential importance of insulin and glucose metabolism, the metabolic syndrome, and diabetes. This raised many questions. Among them were why lack of exercise and obesity should be more likely to lead to central adiposity in South Asians, than in non-Asians.

Diet is an obvious candidate to consider given the differences in average patterns between South Asians and others. The picture is far from clear and will require further examination. One particular hypothesis is that low intake of folic acid in South Asians may account for high levels of plasma homocysteine (see chapter 8 by Sanders in this volume).

The role of infection and inflammation in heart disease in general remains to be clarified. Here, a crucial issue has to do with confounding; might people exposed to infection have been exposed to other adverse environmental conditions?

There is great interest in genetic contributions. These should not be thought of in isolation from environmental influences. For example, twin studies show that obesity is 60 –80% heritable. Yet migrant studies show clear influence of environment. The study comparing Indians in West London with their siblings in India showed a mean difference in body mass index (BMI) of 4. Assuming no difference in height, this corresponds to a mean difference in weight of about 12 kilograms. Putting it differently, it is consistent with an interpretation that people move from the environment where few are overweight (defined as BMI>25) to one where the majority are. The heritability estimates from twin studies understate the contribution of the environment where this changes significantly.

The early life studies sound several cautionary notes (see chapter 5 by Fall in this volume). The high prevalence of low birth weight in India is entirely consistent with the prediction of high rates of heart disease in those birth cohorts. The addition of obesity in childhood and young adulthood is likely to exacerbate that risk. The interaction of influences from early life with circumstance in adulthood will be a fertile area for further research that will be crucial in laying a basis for prevention.

My own early studies of immigrants from the Indian subcontinent suggested very little social gradient in CHD while much of my other research has pointed to the importance of social and psychosocial influences on CHD, which did not seem promising as explanations for the high rate of CHD in South Asians[3]. Williams and Harding argue convincingly that it is time to examine these hypotheses again (see chapter 12 in this volume). Recent data show that there is an inverse social gradient in CHD in South Asians and there may well be an adverse pattern of exposure to psychosocial factors[4].

Although this collection of papers has focussed on coronary heart disease in South Asians there is potentially much to learn from comparisons with other ethnic groups. These can potentially shed light on the way that social and biological factors interact to cause variation in disease rates. This is an area of research that holds much promise for scientific advance. The opportunity should be grasped.

References

1.   Health Survey for England: the health of minority ethnic groups 1999, volumes I and II. Erens, B., Primatesta, P., and Prior, G. 2000. London

2.   McKeigue PM, Pierpoint T, Ferrie JE, Marmot MG. Relationship of glucose intolerance and hyperinsulinaemia to body fat pattern in South Asians and Europeans. Diabetologia 1992;35:785-91.

3.   Marmot MG, Adelstein AM, Bulusu L. Lessons from the study of immigrant mortality. Lancet 1984;1:1455-8.

4.   Hemingway H, Whitty CJM, Shipley M, Stansfeld S, Brunner E, Fuhrer R *et al*. Psychosocial risk factors for coronary disease in white, South Asian and Afro-Caribbean civil servants: the WII study. Ethnicity and Disease 2001;11:391-400.